This book is dedicated to my children

Dakotah Weeks Murphree
and
Ridgeway Harris Murphree

You brighten my cloudiest days.

Thanks for your love, patience, and understanding
while I wrote this book. I love you.

Daddy, life is like a book.
You never know what's going to happen
until you turn the next page.

How true, Dakotah. That's why we have no time to lose.
I hope my work helps you enjoy each and every page of your life.

Treating and Beating Anxiety and Depression

with Orthomolecular Medicine

A Guide for Patients

Dr. Rodger H. Murphree II, DC, CNS

Many manufacturers and sellers claim trademarks on their unique products. When these trademarks appear in this book and we are aware of them, we have used initial capital letters (e.g., Prozac) for designation.

Endnotes designated in the text of this book can be found at the end of each corresponding chapter. Starred footnotes can be found at the bottom of the corresponding page. Patient testimonials are based on actual experiences as observed by the author.

ISBN 0972893814

Printed in the United States of America.
Harrison and Hampton Publishing, Inc.
3401 Independence Dr. Suite 121, Birmingham, AL 35209

Distributed by Cardinal Publishers Group
2222 Hillside Ave. Suite 100, Indianapolis, IN 46218
(317) 879-0871

Editing and book design by Betsy Stokes.
Cover design by Mike McCracken at MCDesign.

Set in 10-point Times New Roman

Contact Dr. Murphree
Inquiries concerning content of this book should be addressed to the author at 3401 Independence Dr. Suite 121, Birmingham, AL, 35209. Phone: (205) 879-2383   Fax: (205) 879-2381

Visit us at www.treatingandbeating.com.

This book and the advice given are not intended to take the place of your physician. Please consult with your health care professional before discontinuing any medication.

"I'd rather have a bottle in front of me than a frontal lobotomy!"

Have you ever, like Groucho Marx quipped in the golden age of comedy, found yourself having to choose the lesser between two evils? When you suffer from a mood disorder, your choices can seem bleak: numb the pain with alcohol, mask your symptoms with drugs…the choices get more destructive from there.

If you suffer from anxiety and/or depression, it likely affects every facet of your life. For many, the pain, disappointment, fatigue, and hopelessness slowly consumes every fiber of their being. They may lose their job, marriage, friends, and family relationships as they spiral into an ever deeper abyss. At its worst, the illness can cause such suffering that death is a welcomed option: over 30,000 Americans commit suicide each year.

Effectively treating anxiety and depression can be quite difficult. We've come a long way since the dark ages, when mood disorders were treated with barbaric therapies: brain surgery with no anesthesia, exorcisms, and shamanistic potions. In the late 18th century, however, Dr. Benjamin Rush, the father of American psychiatry, began to assert that mental illness is actually a "disease of the mind" that needed to be treated as such.

Dr. Rush theorized that "madness" was caused by "morbid" qualities in the blood, leading him to conclude that as much as "four-fifths of the blood in the body" should be drawn away. He bled one patient 47 times, removing four gallons of blood over time. He also strapped patients horizontally to a board and spun them around at great speeds. He confined others in his "tranquilizer chair"—which completely immobilized every part of their body for long periods and blocked their sight with a bizarre wooden shroud—while they were doused in ice-cold water.

Insulin was isolated in 1922, and the idea of insulin coma therapy was introduced into psychiatry 11 years later by Austrian psychiatrist Manfred Sackell. The therapy involved depriving a person's brain of glucose (the form of sugar the brain uses to function) in order to elicit a comatose state. Patients were then dramatically reawaken by a sudden injection of glucose. Patients did seem to be calmer afterwards (brain damage can do that). Unfortunately, this new miracle therapy was also associated with a shockingly high mortality rate! Some physicians began to question its merits, and a randomized trial concluded that insulin coma therapy was not effective. It quickly fell out of favor. Whew!

In the early 1900s, frontal lobotomies and electric shock therapy were standard practice. Shock treatment became an overutilized and indeed cruel form of mass mind control for those housed in mental institutions.

Today, individuals who consult a family doctor for anxiety or depression usually receive a prescription antidepressant. This is most often an SSRI (selective serotonin re-uptake inhibitor) such as Prozac, Effexor, Cymbalta, Paxil, Zoloft, Celex, or Lexapro. Prescription antidepressants can provide excellent relief from the symptoms of anxiety and depression. Consequently, millions of Americans have tried them. In fact, prescription antidepressant sales reached a total of $37 billion in 2003, which was $9 million more than was spent that year on treatments for the heart, arteries, and blood pressure. Preschoolers, in fact, are the fastest-growing group of users.[1] In 2000, over one million American children were taking an antidepressant medication.[2]

However, antidepressant and antianxiety drugs are no panacea. Most individuals may initially benefit from taking an antidepressant drug only to find that the positive effects soon wear off. Several studies show that 19–70% of those taking the drugs would do just as well on a placebo![3] And while patients are attempting to correct their mood disorders with prescription drugs (which might or might not be working), they are facing some potential, sometimes serious, side effects. Prozac alone has been associated with over 1,734 suicide deaths and over 28,000 adverse reactions. Prescription antidepressants can cause depression, anxiety, addiction, suicidal tendencies, involuntary muscle spasms, and senility.[4]

Patients suffering from anxiety more than from depression are commonly prescribed one of the benzodiazepines such as Ativan, Xanax, or Klonopin. These medications are associated with numerous unwanted side effects including poor sleep, seizures, mania, depression, suicide, ringing in the ears, amnesia, dizziness, anxiety, disorientation, low blood pressure, nausea, fluid retention, tremors, sexual dysfunction (decreased desire and performance), weakness, somnolence (prolonged drowsiness or a trance-like condition that may continue for days), and headaches. Over 73,000 older adults experience drug induced tardive dyskinesia (uncontrollable shakes). For many, these tremors are permanent.[5]

A BETTER WAY: ORTHOMOLECULAR

Fortunately for those seeking a safer, often more effective treatment for mood disorders, a group of progressive-minded physicians have pioneered orthomolecular medicine. Orthomolecular physicians recognize that in many cases of physiological and psychological disorders, health can be reestablished by properly correcting, or normalizing, the balance of vitamins, minerals, amino acids, and other similar substances within the body. And unlike drug therapy, which attempts to cover-up or at best temporarily relieve symptoms, orthomolecular medicine seeks to find and correct the causes of illness.

In this book, I'll show you how to discover and treat the physical illness causing your symptoms. I'll present scientific studies to demonstrate how mood disorders are aggravated or even caused by certain nutritional needs. I'll take you through a step-by-step program, based on orthomolecular medicine, to beat your anxiety and depression.

You are unique, and your results will vary from another individual's, but positive changes can be quick and often dramatic. Orthomolecular physicians have helped millions of patients around the world. Perhaps it's your turn to be another success story. Don't give up. You can feel better.

1. Hawkins, Beth. "A Pill is not Enough." www.citypages.com (Minneapolis/St. Paul) v. 25, iss. 1225; May 26, 2004.
2. Waters, Rob. "Drug Report Barred by FDA: Scientist Links Antidepressants to Suicide in Kids" *San Francisco Chronicle;* February 1, 2004. (Archived at www.sfgate.com)
3. Laporte, Joan-Ramone, and Figueras, Albert. "Placebo Effects in Psychiatry" *Lancet* 334 (1993):1206–8.
4. Citizens Commission on Human Rights. See www.cchr.org.
5. Wolfe, Sidney, et al. *Worst Pills Best Pills.* Pocket; 1999. (A 2005 printing is now available.)

Table of Contents

1

The Problem Defined

Major depression is the leading cause of
disability in the US. Anxiety disorders, as a group,
are the most common mental illness in America.

In any given twelve-month period, 9.5% of the population—about 18.8 million American adults—suffer from depression,[1] and depression (and related mood disorders) ranks only behind high blood pressure as the most common reason people visit their doctors. In the course of a lifetime, one out of every four women and one out of every ten men will develop it.[2] Estimates of the direct and indirect annual costs of depression range up to $43 billion.

Although men are only half as likely as women to suffer from depression, at least 3 million men in the United States are affected by the illness. Men are less likely to admit to depression, and doctors are less likely to suspect it in their male patients. Of course, millions of people of both genders go undiagnosed but suffer none the less.

It's not unusual for people to experience periodic low moods associated with the ups and downs of life. Those with clinical depression, however, suffer from a disease process that negatively impacts every facet of life. Their illness is as painful as any physical malady, and it can be just as life threatening. We now know that those with major depression are more likely to suffer a heart attack than those without.[3] Just as dangerous is depression's well-known link to suicide.

DEPRESSIVE DISORDERS

Clinical depression is broken down into three types:

1. Major depression manifests a combination of symptoms that interfere with the ability to work, study, sleep, eat, and enjoy once pleasurable activities. Such a disabling episode of depression may occur only once but more commonly occurs several times in a lifetime.

2. Dysthymia, a less severe type of depression, involves long-term, chronic symptoms that are not disabling but keep someone from functioning well or feeling good. Many people with dysthymia also experience some episodes of major depression.

3. Bipolar disorder is also called manic-depressive disorder. Not nearly as prevalent as other forms of depressive disorders, bipolar disorder is characterized by cyclic mood changes: severe highs (mania) and lows (depression). Sometimes the mood switches are dramatic and rapid, but more often they are gradual. When in the depressed cycle, an individual can have any or all of the symptoms of depression. When in the manic cycle, the individual may be overactive, over-talkative, and wildly energetic. Mania often affects thinking, judgment, and social behavior in ways that cause embarrassment and serious problems. For example, the individual in a manic phase may feel elated, full of grand schemes that might range from unwise business decisions to romantic sprees. Mania, left untreated, can worsen to a psychotic state.

SYMPTOMS OF DEPRESSION AND MANIA

Not everyone who is depressed or manic experiences every symptom listed below. Some people experience a few symptoms; others many. The severity of symptoms varies among individuals and can also fluctuate over time.

SYMPTOMS OF DEPRESSION

- persistent sad, anxious, or "empty" mood
- feelings of hopelessness; pessimism
- feelings of guilt, worthlessness, or helplessness
- loss of interest or pleasure in hobbies and activities that were once enjoyed, including sex
- fatigue, decreased energy, or a feeling of being "slowed down"
- difficulty concentrating, remembering, or making decisions

- insomnia, early-morning wakening, or oversleeping
- loss of appetite and/or weight; overeating or weight gain
- thoughts of death or suicide; suicide attempts
- restlessness or irritability
- persistent physical symptoms that do not respond to treatment, such as headaches, digestive disorders, or chronic pain

SYMPTOMS OF MANIA

- abnormal or excessive elation
- unusual irritability
- decreased need for sleep
- grandiose notions
- increased talking
- racing thoughts
- increased sexual desire
- markedly increased energy
- poor judgment
- inappropriate social behavior

ANXIETY DISORDERS

Often accompanying depression, anxiety disorders are debilitating illnesses that affect more than 19 million American adults each year. Children and adolescents can also develop anxiety disorders.

1. **Panic disorder** involves repeated episodes of intense fear that strike often and without warning. Physical symptoms include chest pain, heart palpitations, shortness of breath, dizziness, abdominal distress, feelings of unreality, and fear of dying.

2. **Obsessive-compulsive disorder** manifests as repeated, unwanted thoughts or compulsive behaviors that seem impossible to stop or control.

3. **Post-traumatic stress disorder** can occur after experiencing or witnessing a traumatic event such as rape or other criminal assault, war, child abuse, natural or human-caused disasters, or automobile crashes. Common symptoms include nightmares, flashbacks, numbing of emotions, depression, anger, irritability, feeling distracted, and being easily startled. Family members of victims can also develop this disorder.

4. Phobias include two major types: social phobia and specific phobia. People with social phobia have an overwhelming and disabling fear of scrutiny, embarrassment, or humiliation in social situations, which leads to avoidance of many potentially pleasurable and meaningful activities. People with specific phobia experience extreme, disabling, and irrational fear of something that poses little or no actual danger; the fear leads to avoidance of objects or situations and can cause people to limit their lives unnecessarily.

5. Generalized anxiety disorder is marked by constant, exaggerated worrisome thoughts and tension about everyday routine life events and activities. These thoughts last at least six months and can be accompanied by physical symptoms such as fatigue, trembling, muscle tension, headache, and nausea.

1.Lee Robins, PhD, and Darrel Regier, MD, MPH (Eds). *Psychiatric Disorders in America: The Epidemiologic Catchment Area Study.* 1990: Free Press.
2.Blehar MD, Oren DA. "Gender differences in depression." *Medscape Women's Health,* 1997;2:3. Revised from: "Women's increased vulnerability to mood disorders: Integrating psychobiology and epidemiology." *Depression,* 1995;3:3-12.
3.KRR Krishnan. "Depression as a contributing factor in cerebrovascular disease." *American Heart Journal,* 2000, Vol 140, Iss 4, Suppl. S, pp 570-576.

2

Feeding Your Brain

Most of what scientists know about the

role our brains play in our moods and behavior is

based on our understanding of *neurotransmitters.*

Also known as monoamines, neurotransmitters are brain chemicals that help relay electrical messages from one nerve cell to another. Examples of neurotransmitters include norepinephrine, dopamine, gamma amino butyric acid (GABA), and the most commonly known: serotonin.

These chemicals are how the brain communicates with itself, to put it simply. Our brains orchestrate our infinite bodily functions through the use of electrochemical "messages" that flow from one neuron (nerve cell) to another. We are born with over one hundred billion neurons, and each one has thousands of finger-like projections that lie next to other neurons but do not touch them. The tiny space between neurons is called the synaptic gap. (We have over one hundred trillion of these neuron-to-neuron gaps.) Nerve cells communicate by using neurotransmitters to bridge these synaptic gaps, allowing electrical brain messages to travel from one neuron to another.

The brain uses electrical charges to monitor all aspects of the body, including heart rate, blood pressure, breathing, movement, and the experience of pain, sadness, happiness, and joy. In this way, our neurotransmitters help regulate pain, reduce anxiety, promote happiness, initiate deep sleep, and boost energy and mental clarity.

Modern antidepressant drug therapy seeks to manipulate the neurotransmitter–synaptic gap interaction. The most popular antidepressants increase the amount of time that neurotransmitters are held within the gap. They are called re-uptake inhibitors, because they inhibit the body's natural ability to "take back up" the neurotransmitter that's in the synaptic gap. This, in theory, increases the availability of the neurotransmitters so that they can be used more effectively by the brain. To help you understand this concept, picture someone using a gasoline additive to get more mileage from the gas in her car.

Sounds like a good idea, right? Well, although adding a gasoline additive to your tank might help for a time, sooner or later, you could still be running on empty. Then there won't be any gasoline to augment (serotonin to re-uptake) in her tank (brain). Using a gasoline additive won't help if you have a gasoline deficiency. In the same way, you might be suffering from a serotonin deficiency, and inhibiting re-uptake all day won't help.

The good news is that we now know what raw materials the body uses to create the neurotransmitters! Certain vitamins, minerals, essential fatty acids, and amino acids are used to build the brain chemicals we need. For instance, the amino acid tryptophan turns into serotonin. So a safe, natural, and highly successful approach to increasing serotonin levels involves supplementing with the amino acid tryptophan. Do you see the connection? There is no need to use a gasoline additive when you can simply add more gasoline to the tank! By taking the appropriate amino acid and its synergistic vitamins and minerals, you can help your body create it's own, natural, necessary neurotransmitters.

This treatment not only applies to serotonin deficiencies. Some individuals might be taking an antidepressant designed to boost epinephrine levels (such as Effexor, Cymbalta, or Wellbutren). But the natural amino acid phenylalanine, plus certain synergistic vitamins and minerals, is responsible for making epinephrine. So why take a drug associated with numerous side effects when you can use the natural raw ingredient that actually makes the chemical you need? Amino acid replacement therapy is at least as effective as prescription antidepressants, and amino acid replacement therapy has few, if any, side effects.[1]

NEUROTRANSMITTERS

- **Serotonin,** created from the amino acid tryptophan, elevates mood, reduces food cravings, reduces pain, increases mental clarity, reduces IBS symptoms, promotes deep sleep, relieves tension, and calms the body.

- **Dopamine and norepinephrine** are synthesized from the amino acid phenylalanine. They increase mental and physical alertness, reduce fatigue, and elevate mood.

- **Epinephrine** is a neurotransmitter that helps increase energy and boost mental clarity. When low, it causes depression and fatigue. Prescription medications like Wellbutrin and Effexor attempt to boost the brain's level of epinephrine. However, a person can easily increase his epinephrine levels naturally.

- **Gamma-aminobutyric acid (GABA)** is a tripeptide made from three amino acids. It has a calming effect on the brain similar to that of Valium and other tranquilizers without the side effects. GABA, used in combination with the B vitamins niacinamide (a form of B3) and inositol, can alleviate anxiety and panic attacks. Many of my patients are surprised by the effectiveness of GABA in treating their anxiety and panic attacks.

Neurotransmitters that cause excitatory and stimulating reactions are known as catecholamines. These include epinephrine and norepinephrine (adrenaline). Inhibitory or relaxing neurotransmitters include serotonin and gamma-aminobutyric acid (GABA).

AMINO ACIDS

There are 20 amino acids. Nine are known as essential amino acids. They can't be made by the body and must be obtained from our diet. Non-essential amino acids can be manufactured from within our own cells. See the chart on the top of the facing page.

ESSENTIAL

- isoleucine
- leucine
- lysine
- methionine
- phenylalanine
- threonine
- tryptophan
- valine
- histadine

NON-ESSENTIAL

- glycine
- glutamic acid
- arginine
- aspartic acid
- alanine
- proline
- serine
- tyrosine
- cysteine
- glutamine
- asparagine

Amino acids are involved in every bodily function. They are the raw materials for the reproduction and growth of every cell. They are in every bone, organ (including the brain), muscle, and most every hormone.

Individual amino acids are joined together in sequential chains to form proteins. Protein, the body's building material, is essential to every cell and makes up our muscles, hair, bones, collagen, and connective tissue. Enzymes are protein molecules that coordinate thousands of chemical reactions taking place in the body. They are essential for breaking down and digesting our food.

Amino acids can occur in two forms: D-form and L-form, which are mirror images of one another. The L-form is available in the foods we eat and is considered the more absorbable. D-forms can be created by bacteria, tissue catabolism, or synthetic means. Most D-form amino acids are not available for protein synthesis and can be detrimental to normal enzyme functions. DL-phenylalanine, however, is the exception. DL-phenylalanine is good for you, inhibiting the breakdown of endorphins and enkephalin, which elevate mood and help block pain. These are the same chemicals released during strenuous exercise to create the "runner's high."

DISORDERS OF AMINO ACID DEFICIENCIES[2]

- fatigue
- depression
- anxiety
- mental confusion
- chemical sensitivities
- dermatitis
- cardiovascular disease

- high blood pressure
- inflammatory disorders
- poor detoxification
- insomnia
- osteoporosis
- poor immunity
- arthritis

HOW TO SUPPLEMENT WITH AMINO ACIDS

Always use the L forms of an amino acid when supplementing. Amino acids can be taken as a blend to shore up any nutritional deficiencies or taken individually in order to produce specific reactions. It's best to take single amino acids on an empty stomach, 30 minutes before or 1 hour after eating. Individuals with malabsorption syndrome, irritable bowel, leaky gut, and chronic illnesses are wise to take an amino acid blend in addition to any single amino acids they may be taking.

I've treated thousands of patients with mood disorders and have been using amino acid replacement therapy for several years. I've found this approach to be far superior to prescription medicines (in most cases) for treating mild to moderate mood disorders. I've found very few problems with mixing the recommended supplements with prescription antidepressants. However, I advise you to seek the advice of a health professional is familiar with orthomolecular medicine, if possible.

There are various questionnaires and self-tests available, developed by myself and others, to help you determine which amino acids you need. In chapter 5, you'll get started with my Brain Function Questionnaire.

1.Bressa, G.M. "S-Adenosyl-l-methionine (SAMe) as antidepressant: meta-analysis of clinical studies." *Acta Neurol. Scand. Suppl.* 1994; 154: 7–14.
2.Great Smokies Diagnostic Laboratory *Application Guide for Physicians*

3

Dangers of Drug Treatment

Antidepressants can cause depression, anxiety,
addiction, suicidal tendencies, debilitating muscle
spasms, and dementia. And our most vulnerable —
children and the elderly — are the most in danger.

In 1954, the sedative Thorazine (chlorpromazine), fueled by a huge
promotion campaign, swept the nation and spawned an entirely new
class of drugs: **tranquilizers.** Thought to induce a "chemical loboto-
my," Thorazine became the drug *du jour* of the 1950s (much like Prozac
and other SSRIs are today) as the number of individuals taking
Thorazine rocketed from 428 in 1952 to over 2,000,000 in 1957.[1]

Thorazine and similar tranquilizers were frequently recommended for
any number of illnesses associated with mental stress (before Thorazine,
alcohol and opiates had been the treatments of choice). In the 1960s,
Hoffman La Roche successfully marketed the benzodiazepine tranquilizers Librium and Valium. Aggressive marketing resulted in physicians
prescribing these medications for a number of unrelated illnesses including asthma, high blood pressure, and ulcers. To combat the ills of
modern-day stress, housewives, college students, and busy executives
were encouraged to try a tranquilizer. Valium became America's best-
selling drug, and eventually, over 250 million people worldwide had
taken a tranquilizer.[2] Unfortunately, quite a number of potential side
effects are associated with these medications: confusion, lethargy,

memory impairment, tics (uncontrollable muscle spasms), parkinsonism, agitation, depression, and addiction. By 1977, neurological testing had shown that up to 40% of those taking tranquilizers had developed uncontrollable twitching.[3] Not surprisingly, the public at large began to become disenchanted with this class of drugs. It didn't take long before the pharmaceutical industry came up with another "new and better" solution to depression.

The modern era of antidepressant medication began with the discovery of **tricyclic antidepressant (TCA)** drugs. Named for their three-ringed chemical structure, TCAs block the re-uptake by the brain of norepinephrine and serotonin. They can be effective in relieving anxiety and, to a lesser extent, depression, but they have an overall sedating effect that tends to mask all emotions. The first TCA was Tofranil (imipramine), originally developed in 1957 in search of a treatment for schizophrenia. Although ineffective for its original use, it appeared to elevate the moods of patients with major depression while merely sedating those without it. This led to the idea that Tofranil was selectively reversing depression and not, like the older tranquilizers, merely producing a generalized sedation.

In the 1960s, Merck introduced amitriptyline (Elavil), which soon became the most popular TCA. But in their fervor, Merck not only promoted amitriptyline but depression as well. Up until the popularization of these newer medications, depression was thought to affect 50–100 people per million. Recent estimates, however, put that number at 100,000 per million; that's a thousand-fold increase!

Other examples of TCAs include Endep, Vanatrip, Asendin, Anafranil, Norpramin, Adapin, Sinequan, Aventyl, Pamelor, and Vivactil. Like other antidepressant medications, these drugs are processed by the liver and can cause liver toxicity. Common side effects include sedation, confusion, blurred vision, weight gain (Elavil is especially notorious), muscle spasms or tremors, dry mouth, convulsions, constipation, difficulty in urinating, and sensitivity to light. Talk about depressing!

Developed soon afterwards, **monoamine oxidase inhibitor (MAOI)** drugs bring about similar results as TCAs but work by blocking an enzyme called monoamine oxidase. Turning off the MAO enzyme allows more of the neurotransmitters (for example, serotonin and norepinephrine) to be left in the synaptic gaps of the brain for longer periods. Unfortunately, MAOIs also prevent the breakdown of an amino acid known as tyramine. Buildup of tyramine can contribute to high blood pressure, which could lead to stroke, heart attack, and other side effects. Consequently people using MAOIs must avoid foods high in tyramine: alcohol, legumes, cheese, fish, ginseng, meat, sauerkraut, shrimp paste, soups, and yeast extracts. These dietary restrictions can present major complications for patients.

Though still in limited use today, TCAs and MAOIs have been eclipsed by the newer and largely overhyped **selective serotonin re-uptake inhibitors (SSRIs).** The first SSRI to hit the American market was Prozac, in 1987.

PROZAC AND OTHER SSRIs

Prozac was cleared by the FDA in 1988 and by 1994 had become the fastest growing prescription drug in America, with sales over $1.2 billion. Two other SSRI drugs, Paxil and Zoloft, have seen similar success. In 1998 these three medications accounted for over $4 billion in annual sales. As many as 10% of the US population have at one time or another taken an SSRI drug.

Within two years of its debut, Prozac was the number one antidepressant drug. *New York* magazine called it a "wonder drug." In March 1990, it graced the cover of *Newsweek,* which hailed it as a "medical breakthrough" and reported that "even healthy people have started asking for it."

In 1993, psychiatrist Peter Kramer released his book *Listening to Prozac,* filled with unsubstantiated, over-the-top reports of the drug's benefits. Kramer suggested that if you didn't like your personality, you could always choose to improve it by "cosmetic psychopharmacology." This book helped spread the myth of the "miracle" of Prozac and other SSRIs. Soon, primary care physicians, *not* psychiatrists, were writing 70% of all SSRI prescriptions.[4]

Why were SSRIs like Prozac so celebrated? For one thing, they were believed to be safer and more effective than TCAs or MAOIs. Similar to these older drugs, SSRIs block the reuptake of serotonin within the synaptic gap. But SSRIs are more selective, affecting serotonin while leaving other brain chemicals alone. This theoretically minimizes the more serious side effects of TCAs and MAOIs.

But in the rush to promote these "wonder drugs" for a variety of illnesses including headaches, PMS, menopause, chronic pain, obsessive compulsive disorder, and of course anxiety and depression, the potential side effects of SSRIs have been rarely mentioned. In fact, the success of SSRIs is largely due to the false belief that they pose relatively few risks. Dr. Kramer has helped promote this idea by writing such statements as, "There is no unhappy ending to this story."

However, like most miracle cures, panaceas and drugs *du jour,* there has been a growing backlash to Prozac, as it has become associated with over 1,734 suicide deaths and over 28,000 adverse reactions.[5]

THE UNTOLD RISKS

Prescription drugs have helped millions of people overcome mental illnesses and mood disorders, and antidepressants are sometimes helpful for my patients. But make no mistake: they don't correct the problem. My patients don't come to me with a Prozac deficiency, so pumping in Prozac isn't the solution.

Plus, the side effects of these drugs can cause an assortment of health problems. Prescription antidepressants can cause depression, anxiety, addiction, suicidal tendencies, tardive dyskinesia (involuntary muscle spasms), and tardive dementia (senility).[6] You read that right. Prescription antidepressants and anti-anxiety drugs can and do cause depression and anxiety.

Children, especially, are susceptible to the most dangerous aspects of antidepressant therapy. Still, young children are often prescribed psychotropic drugs for pain relief, anxiety, bed wetting, and ADD/ADHD disorder. The number of 2–4-year-olds on psychiatric drugs (including Ritalin) and antidepressants (such as Prozac) jumped 50 percent from 1991 to 1995.[7] And this trend has not slowed. In fact, the largest growth spurt in antidepressant use has been among preschoolers.[8] The use of antidepressants and other psychiatric medication among children has more than tripled in recent years and now approaches adult usage rates, according to a January 2003 study in the *Archives of Pediatric and Adolescent Medicine.*

Just last year, FDA medical officer and child psychiatrist Andrew Mosholder reviewed data from 20 clinical trials involving more than 4,100 children and eight different antidepressants. He concluded that there was an increased risk of suicidal behavior among children being treated for depression with antidepressants.[9]

BUT AREN'T SSRIs SAFE?

Though SSRI drugs are a great improvement over their predecessors, many scientists are advocating a closer investigation of their potential dangers. Consider the following from Dr. Candace Pert, the scientist who helped uncover the interaction of drugs and neurotransmitters:

> "I am alarmed at the monster that Johns Hopkins neuroscientist Solomon Snyder and I created when we discovered the simple binding assay for drug receptors 25 years ago. Prozac and other antidepressant serotonin-receptor-active compounds may also cause cardiovascular problems in some susceptible people after long-term use, which has become common practice despite the lack of safety studies.
>
> "The public is being misinformed about the precision of these selective serotonin-uptake inhibitors when the medical profession oversimplifies their action in the brain and ignores the body as if it exists merely to carry the head around! In short, these molecules of emotion regulate every aspect of our physiology. A new paradigm has evolved, with implications that life-style changes such as diet and exercise can offer profound, safe and natural mood elevation."[10]

Common side effects of SSRIs include headache, muscle pain, chest pain, anxiety, nervousness, sleeplessness, drowsiness, weakness, changes in sex drive, tremors, dry mouth, irritated stomach, loss of appetite, dizziness, nausea, rash, itching, weight gain, diarrhea, impotence, hair loss, dry skin, chest pain, bronchitis, abnormal heart beat, twitching, anemia, low blood sugar, and low thyroid.[11]

These adverse side effects are more common than most patients will admit and and most doctors are aware. Doctors simply don't suspect that their patients' bronchitis, irritable bowel syndrome, fatigue, or low thyroid is a result of taking SSRI drugs. Instead when a patient presents with chest pain, he's referred to a cardiologist for a battery of tests, which usually come back normal. The cardiologist might prescribe a drug to help with the chest pain—perhaps a beta blocker like Toprol. This brings the patient only fatigue and more depression. Once back at the psychiatrist's office, he is given Wellbutrin to boost his energy. The patient may then have problems falling asleep, so his family doctor prescribes Ambien, which can cause short-term memory loss and further depression. And so the cycle feeds itself. Meanwhile none of the consulting doctors ever suspects the initial SSRI drug as the originator of the problem. Tragically, this scenario is all too common.

THE NEXT LEVEL: SSNRIs

Effexor (venlafaxine) and the newer Cymbalta (duloxetine) are selective serotonin and norepinephrine re-uptake inhibitor drugs (SSNRIs). They can cause dizziness, fatigue, loss of libido, dry mouth, stomach pain, indigestion, high blood pressure, nervousness, anxiety, tingling or loss of feeling in the hands or toes, chest pain, seizures, breathing difficulties, diarrhea, lightheadedness, fainting, headache, lockjaw, menstrual changes, depression, restlessness, ringing in the ears, swelling in legs or feet, and vision changes.[12]

The January 2005 issue of *Best Pills Worst Pills News* reports that Cymbalta (duloxetine) has been shown to cause liver toxicity.[13] It can also cause high blood pressure. Cymbalta has been marketed as an anti-depressant that also helps block pain, but *The Medical Letter on Drugs and Therapeutics* found that Cymbalta was "nothing special" and con-cluded their October 11, 2004 report by saying: "Whether duloxetine offers any advantage over venlafaxine or an SSRI like fluoxetine remains to be established. The manufacturer's claim that duloxetine is the antidepressant for painful symptoms associated with depression is unsupported—no comparative trials are available."[14]

Cymbalta has been aggressively marketed as a treatment for fibromyal-gia.* Some of my fibromyalgia patients have been duped into taking Cymbalta without realizing that this medication may actually make their condition worse. A number of them have reported to me that Cymbalta caused them to experience dizziness, anxiety, chest pain, and breathing problems, for which they were unprepared.

Doctors are supposed to warn their patients about the potential side effects of any drugs they recommend! But when was the last time your doctor went into detail about the possible side effects of a prescription antidepressant? Sadly, in my experience, it just doesn't happen.

---

*Fibromyalgia, a syndrome identified by diffuse muscle pain, poor sleep, depression, anxiety, and other problems, is discussed in detail in my earlier book, *Treating and Beating Fibromyalgia and Chronic Fatigue Syndrome.*

ATYPICAL ANTIDEPRESSANTS

Somewhat in a class of their own are Desyrel (trazadone) and Wellbutrin (buproprion). Desyrel blocks serotonin uptake, is very sedating, and is often used to treat sleep disorders. It can cause dizziness, fainting, cardiac arrhythmias, low blood pressure, overstimulation, headaches, fatigue, nausea, impotence, seizures, and altered liver function.

Wellbutrin increases norepinephrine and dopamine levels. It can cause agitation, seizures, insomnia, tremors, dry mouth, headaches, psychosis, migraines, swelling, heart palpitations, urinary frequency, sweating, and ringing in the ears. Do these sound like drugs you really want to be taking?

THE EXPENSIVE PLACEBO

Some folks decide that suffering the side effects and unknown dangers of antidepressants is worth the risk for the benefit achieved. But what if you discovered that you would do just as well taking a sugar pill (with the only potential side effect being tooth decay)? Studies have shown just that. In fact, between 19-70% of those taking antidepressant medications do just as well taking a placebo.[15]

A recent meta-analysis of published clinical trials indicates that 75% of the response to antidepressants is duplicated by placebo.[16] In other words, real prescription antidepressants may only be a little more effective than fake ones in relieving the symptoms of anxiety and depression. Combine this fact with the drug's potential side effects, and the idea of using drugs to cover up your symptoms becomes less appealing. It's just not worth it, even when it works.

SOME SIDE EFFECTS OF SSRIs

- **Link to suicide:** As discussed earlier, SSRI use has been linked to an increased risk of suicide in teenagers and children. Drug regulators have recommended that Paxil not be newly prescribed to anyone under age 18. Some regulators believe the risk extends to adult patients, as well.[17]

- **Decreased libido:** The insert data for most SSRI antidepressant medications report that only 2–4% of those taking these drugs experience decreased libido. However, this report is scandalously low. In my experience, the majority of men and especially women taking SSRIs suffer from low libido. Numerous studies show that as many as 86% suffer from sexual dysfunction.[18]

- **Weight gain or unhealthy loss:** My patients on Prozac will often complain that their senses of smell and taste have decreased, causing a lost interest in food. And some diet centers use Prozac as an appetite suppressant. More than one patient has shared that once she discontinued taking Prozac, she gained back her lost weight and then some. The other SSRI medications are all associated with weight gain, and Paxil seems to be the worst culprit. I've had several patients who've gained 30–40 pounds in a single year after starting Paxil.[19]

- **Tics:** All of the SSRI drugs have been found to possibly cause involuntary muscle twitches called tics (or tardive dyskinesia). These occur in just a few people, but if you're in the lucky 1–2%, the statistics won't matter to you. Tics are simply horrendous. In one especially dramatic case reported in *The American Journal of Psychiatry,* a patient who had recently started Prozac was soon plagued with a nightmarish tic. She was unable to control her tongue, which darted back and forth across her teeth, accompanied by intermittent jaw clinching and sucking in of her cheeks. When she discontinued Prozac, her tics subsided but never totally stopped.[20]

- **Muscle spasms:** General muscle spasms are more common than tics in SSRI users. These spasms often occur in the neck, shoulders, or low back and can greatly complicate the conditions of fibromyalgia patients. Some of these SSRI-induced muscle spasms can be quite dramatic, such as lockjaw and severe torticollis (frozen-stiff neck muscles).[21]

- **Depression:** The numbing of all senses and the dulling of personality and creativity is not uncommon in those taking SSRI medications. And so, many of the drugs used to treat anxiety and depression may in fact cause anxiety and depression. The initial insert for Prozac stated that "depression" was "frequently" reported as an adverse effect of the drug. Not surprisingly, manufacturer Eli Lilly decided to edit this statement at the last minute.[22]

SIDE EFFECTS OF ANTI-ANXIETY DRUGS

Benzodiazepine drugs, usually used to treat anxiety or as "sleeping pills," include Xanax, Klonopin, Ativan, Restoril, BuSpar, Tranxene,

Serax, Librium, Tegretol, Valium, Trileptal, Seroquel, Risperdal, and Symbyax. They all can be addictive, and patients can build up a tolerance so that the drug eventually loses it effectiveness, especially if it's used as a sleep aid. Two million Americans are addicted to minor tranquilizers or sleeping pills, and 15,000 Americans die from sleeping pills each year.[23]

Side effects associated with these medications include poor sleep, seizures, neuropsychiatric disturbances (mania, depression, thoughts of suicide, etc.), tinnitus (ringing in the ears), transient memory loss (amnesia), dizziness, anxiety, disorientation, hypotension (low blood pressure), nausea, edema (fluid retention), ataxia (muscular incoordination), tremors, sexual dysfunction (decreased desire and performance), asthenia (weakness), somnolence (prolonged drowsiness or a trance-like condition that can continue for days), and headaches.

Benzodiazepine medications are also notorious for causing tics and tremors, especially in older adults. Over 73,000 seniors experience some type of drug-induced tics or tremors, and for many these effects are permanent.[24] In fact, 40% of those age 60 or older who take tranquilizers will experience tics.[25] And over 163,000 older Americans experience serious mental impairment (dementia, memory loss, etc.) from taking tranquilizers or sleeping pills.[26] These side effects can also lead to accidents. Each year, over 32,000 older Americans taking tranquilizers fall and break a hip. And tranquilizers and tricyclic antidepressants are the cause of untold numbers of other accidents, including automobile collisions that can claim innocent lives.[27]

With 5.6 million adults over the age of 65 taking tranquilizers,[28] is it any wonder we have so many elderly with pre-senile dementia, Parkinson-like symptoms, mood disorders, fatigue, lethargy, and tremors?

OTHER MEDICATIONS

Many common prescription medications can also cause depression. These include blood pressure medicines such as beta blockers (including Atenolol, Nadolol, and Propranolol), diuretics, the H2 receptor antagonist types of ulcer medication (including Nizatidine, Cimetidine, Famotidine, and Ranitidine), Neurontin, steroids (such as prednisone), oral contraceptives and other artificial female hormones, muscle relaxants, and chemotherapy agents.[29] Many other medications can cause or exacerbate depression or anxiety. Be sure to look up all of your current medications in the Physicians' Desk Reference (PDR) or at www.pdrhealth.com to check on potential side effects.

ENDING DRUG THERAPY

The effects of these drugs on your body is intense, and discontinuing any medication can be equally so. Never discontinue any medication before discussing it with your medical doctor, and always follow his guidelines for doing so. In addition, I don't recommend you stop taking your prescription medications until after you start feeling better on my program. Start taking the supplements I recommend, build up your stress-coping system, and allow your body to start healing itself. After you start feeling stronger (it may take a few months), and with your doctor's help, slowly wean off the medications.

You may still experience withdrawal symptoms with certain medications, so they might need to be restarted until you become stronger or find other less toxic options. Give yourself at least two months to wean off an antidepressant and two–three months to wean off a benzodiazepine drug. Some antidepressant-related withdrawal symptoms can last up to three months after discontinuing the medication. Withdrawal symptoms of benzodiazepines can last up to one year.

Watch for these possible withdrawal symptoms: severe depression, anxiety, agitation, dizziness, a spinning sensation, swaying, difficulty walking, nausea, vomiting, upset stomach, flu-like symptoms, lethargy, muscle pain, tingling, electric shock sensations, and sleep disturbances. (To reduce tremors associated with withdrawal, try taking an additional 50–100 mg. of zinc daily. This is a tip from another orthomolecular physician, and I've found it to be helpful. I also recommend adding up to a gram of manganese with the zinc to get the best results.) You might conclude that your withdrawal symptoms of depression and/or anxiety are because you still need the mood disorder drug. However, this is often not the case. Like an alcoholic who stops drinking, you might have to feel worse before you feel better.

1.(Figures from Judith Swazey's book *Chlorpromazine in Psychiatry* published 1974.)

2.F.J. Ayd, "Prevention of Recurrence (Maintenance Therapy)," in A. DiMascio and R.I. Shader, eds., *Clinical Handbook of Pharmacology* (New York: Science House, 1970), pp.297-310.

3.G.m. Asnis, M.A. Leopold, R.C. Duvoisin, and A.H. Schwartz, "A Survey of Tardive Dyskinesia (tics) in Psychiatric Outpatients," *American Journal of Psychiatry* 134 (1977):136-70

4.M.J. Grinfeld, "Protecting Prozac," *California Lawyer,* December 1998, pp36-40, 79.

5."Death and near death attributed to Prozac." Citizens Commission on Human Rights. See also Whittle TJ, Wiland Richard, "The story behind Prozac the killer drug," *Freedom Magazine,* 6331 Hollywood BLVD., suite 1200 Los Angeles, CA 90028.

6.*Monthly Prescribing Reference* Haymarket Media Publication Nov 2005, New York NY

7.*JAMA* February 23, 2000;283:1025-1030,1059-1060

8.Beth Hawkins, "A Pill is not Enough" City Pages.com Vol 25 issue 1225 Minneapolis MN

9.Rob Waters "Drug Report Barred by FDA: Scientist Links Antidepressants to Suicide in Kids" *San Francisco Chronicle* February 1, 2004. (Archived at www.sfgate.com)

10.Candace B. Pert, Research Professor, Georgetown University Medical Center, Washington; Letter to the Editor of *TIME* Magazine, October 20, 1997, page 8.

11.See 6 above.

12.Sidney Wolfe, Larry Sasich, and Rose-Ellen Hope, *Worst Pills Best Pills.* Pocket Books New York, NY 1999.

13.ibid.

14.ibid.

15.Joan-Ramone Laporte and Albert Figueras, "Placebo Effects in Psychiatry," *Lancet* 334 (1993):1206-8.

16.Kirsch, I., & Sapirstein, G. (1998). "Listening to Prozac but hearing placebo: A meta analysis of antidepressant medication." *Prevention & Treatment,* 1, Article 0002a.

17.FDA *Talk Paper* T04-31 August 20, 2004.

18.J.G. Modell, C.R. Katholi, J.D. Modell and R.L. DePalma, "Comparative Sexual Side Effects of Buprpion (Wellbutrin), Fluoxentine (Prozac), Paroxetine (Paxil), and Sertraline (Zoloft)," *Clinical Pharmacology and Therapeutics* 61 (1997):476-87.

19.Fava M, Judge R, Hoog SL, Nilsson ME, Koke SC. "Fluoxetine versus sertraline and paroxetine in major depressive disorder: changes in weight with long-term treatment." *J Clin Psychiatry.* 2000 Nov;61(11):863-7.

20.C.L Budman and R.D. Bruun, "Persistent Dyskinesia (tics) in a Patient Receiving Fluoxetine (Prozac)," *American Journal of Psychiatry* 148 (1991): 1403.

21.H.Y. Meltzer, M. Young, J. Metz, V.S. Fang, P.S. Schyve, and R.C. Aroroa, "Extrapyramidal Side Effects and Increased Serum Prolactin Following Fluoxetine, a New Antidepressant, " *Journal of Neural Transmission* 45 (1979):165-75

22.Peter Breggin and David Cohen. *Your Drug May Be Your Problem,* De Capo Press, Cambridge MA 2000. p.54.

23.Drs. Peter M. Brooks and Richard O. Day, *New Eng J of Med,* 1991;324(24): 1716–25.

24.See 12 above.

25.Evans LK. "Sundown syndrome in institutional elderly." *Journal of the American Geriatrics Society.* 1987; 35:101-8.

26.Larson EB, Kukull WA, Buchner D, Reifler BV. "Adverse drug reactions associated with global cognitive impairment in elderly persons." *Annals of Internal Medicine* 1987; 107:169-73.

27.See 12 above.

28.See 12 above.

29.A.F. Schatzberg, P. Haddad, E.M. Kaplan, M. Lejoyeux, J.F. Rosenbaum, A.H. Young, and J. Zajecka, "Serotonin Reuptake Inhibitor Discontinuation Syndrome: A Hypothetical Definition" *Journal of Clin Psych* 58 (1997) (suppl.7): 5-10.

4

Your Body is its
Best Healer

Are you convinced yet that drugs are not the answer?
They are very seldom necessary to treat your depression and anxiety, and they can cause a whole lot
more harm than the risk is worth.

Fortunately for those looking for a more natural and often more effective approach, there is orthomolecular medicine. "Ortho" means
correct or normal, and orthomolecular physicians seek to normalize the
body's internal balance.

Like their more conventional colleagues, orthomolecular psychiatrists
acknowledge that mental disorders originate from faulty brain chemistry.
However, they rely less on prescription medications for treatment of
these disorders. They instead recognize the important role that nutrients,
including amino acids, play in creating and regulating neurotransmitters.
They then seek to uncover any nutritional deficiencies that may be causing the mental disorder. Once these deficient nutrients are found, they are
then corrected to optimal levels.

The premise of orthomolecular medicine dates back to the 1920s, when
vitamins and minerals were first used to treat illnesses unrelated to
nutrient deficiency. During that time, it was discovered that vitamin A

could prevent some childhood deaths from infectious illness and that heart arrhythmia (irregular heartbeat) could be stopped by dosages of magnesium. Evidence also began to surface of the benefits of ortho-molecular medicine as a complement to traditional therapies. The studies of Abram Hoffer, MD, and Humphrey Osmond, MD, showed that accompanying their standard medical therapy for schizophrenia with large doses of niacin doubled the number of recoveries they saw in a one-year period.

In 1968, two-time Nobel Prize-winner Linus Pauling, PhD, originated the term "orthomolecular" to describe this approach to medicine. One of the greatest biochemists of the 20th century, this brilliant scientist con-tributed immeasurably to the study of mental illness. He was the first to call mental disorders "molecular diseases" occurring from biochemical abnormalities. He admonished doctors to use the chemicals normally present in the body to treat these abnormalities, insisting that drugs can't replace the nutrients needed for optimal brain function. He fur-thered challenged doctors to investigate and apply the growing amount of data validating the use of megavitamin therapy: "The brain is the most sensitive of all our organs to variations in its molecular composi-tion, and mental symptoms of avitaminosis often are observed long before any physical symptoms appear."[1]

In 1987, Richard Kunin, MD, summarized the principles of orthomole-cular medicine:

1. Nutrition comes first in medical diagnosis and treatment, and nutri-ent-related disorders are usually curable once the nutritional balance is achieved.

2. Biochemical individuality is the norm in medical practice; therefore RDA values are unreliable nutrient guidelines. Many people require an intake of certain nutrients far beyond the RDA suggested range (often called megadoses), due to their genetic disposition, and/or the environment in which they live or work. See more about this in chap-ter 9.

3. Drug treatment is used only for specific indications and always mind-ful of the potential dangers and adverse effects.

4. Environmental pollution and food adulteration are an inescapable fact of modern life and are a medical priority.

5. Blood tests do not necessarily reflect tissue levels of nutrients.

6. Hope is the indispensable ally of the physician and the absolute right of the patient.[2]

TODAY'S RDA: ONE SIZE FAILS ALL

Even with all this progress, many physicians today neglect the role that proper nutrition plays in relation to our health. The prevalent and grossly incorrect notion is that a balanced diet supplies all the nutrients needed for the body to work properly. This draconian thinking flies in the face of the research showing up in our very own medical journals.

Complicating the matter is reliance on the US government's recommended daily allowance (RDA) for proper vitamin and mineral doses. The RDA originated in the 1940s and has had only minor increases since its beginning. Yet individuals in our society are bombarded with over 500 toxic chemicals on a daily basis. Much of our food supply is processed and grown in nutritionally depleted soil. And even if healthy food is available, the majority of American diets are deficient in many vital nutrients, due simply to uninformed or poor food choices.

Although following the RDA may prevent severe deficiency disease, these levels do not provide for optimal health, and people may need many more times the RDA level of certain nutrients. For example, studies of guinea pigs show a 20-fold variation in their requirements for vitamin C. Similar studies in humans have revealed that children have varying needs for vitamin B6.

ARE MEGADOSES SAFE?

One of the arguments against megavitamin treatment is that high doses of certain vitamins are toxic and can cause adverse reactions. Let's investigate the statistics behind this concern: The American Medical Association reports that death from medical errors is now the third leading cause of death in the US (behind heart disease and cancer). Over 250,000 Americans die each year from medical therapies, including at least 113,000 from the negative effects of prescription medications.[3] The total number of deaths from vitamin/mineral therapy during the years of 1983 to 1990 is zero. I like those odds.

Never the less, problems certainly can occur with megavitamin or herbal therapy. When symptoms do arise, however, reducing or stopping the therapy will almost always terminate any side effects. In the 10 years I've been using orthomolecular doses of vitamins, minerals, and amino acids, both intravenously and orally, I have not seen a single major side effect in any of my patients.

IDENTIFYING THE CAUSES

To correct the biochemical deficiencies underlying your mood disorder, we'll need to uncover and correct the causes. Deficiencies can be triggered by any number of chemical, environmental, or emotional stresses.

To help you understand how something like daily stress can actually alter your brain chemistry, visualize a bank savings account statement. We are all born with a "stress-coping" savings account, and the size of this account is largely determined by our genetics. You can't change how you were created; some folks start out with large accounts, and some, small.

But all our accounts are filled with, instead of money, stress-coping chemicals such as serotonin, dopamine, norepinephrine, and cortisol. Every day, we make withdrawals from our account. The more emotional, chemical, mental, and physical stress we encounter, the more withdrawals we need to make. That's OK; that's what the account is there for!

But if you're not careful, and you take out more than you invest in yourself, you can bankrupt your account! This usually leads to fatigue, physical complaints, anxiety, and/or depression. There's no such thing as overdraft protection here! When you don't have enough neurotransmitters and stress-coping chemicals, you simply can't function well.

Poor sleep depletes mood-controlling neurotransmitters including serotonin. Decreased serotonin leads to depression, mental fatigue, lowered pain threshold, and sugar cravings. For more about the dangers of poor sleep, see chapter 6.

Protein deficiencies, due to low-protein diets, poor digestion, or malabsorption syndromes can cause amino acid deficiencies. And amino acids (along with vitamin and mineral cofactors) create the neurotransmitters. Serotonin, for instance, is made from the amino acid tryptophan.

Nutritional deficiencies, you might be surprised to learn, are quite common in America. In one study, up to 50% of patients admitted for hospital care were suffering from nutritional deficiencies.[4] And a deficiency of any of the essential nutrients can create a chain reaction leading to mood disorders, panic disorders, anxiety, and/or depression.

Chromium deficiency, for instance, which is especially common among those taking cholesterol-lowering drugs, can cause hypoglycemia and mood disorders.[5] A deficiency in vitamin C affects production of dopamine, norepinephrine, serotonin, and adrenaline (the fight or flight hormone). Deficient adrenaline levels can lead to fatigue, depression and confusion.

Dopamine, gamma-aminobutyric acid (GABA), and serotonin—all important brain chemicals—rely on magnesium and vitamin B6 for their production. But 50% of the population is deficient in magnesium.[6] And even if you have enough magnesium, if you're on birth control pills or hormone replacement, your medication could be depleting your B6.[7]

Food and chemical sensitivities (allergies) can cause all sorts of symptoms. Allergic inflammation of the mucous membranes of the intestinal tract causes irritable bowel syndrome. Allergic inflammation of the nasal membranes creates sinusitis. Allergic reactions in the respiratory tissue create bronchial spasms (asthma). Allergic reactions can also occur within the brain, creating mental confusion, depression, anxiety, and other mood disorders.

Low thyroid function is associated with stress, depression, anxiety and fatigue. When working properly, thyroid hormones help regulate concentration, mental clarity, moods, and proper brain chemistry. Specifically, the thyroid hormone triiodothyronine (T3) regulates the levels and actions of serotonin, norepinephrine, and GABA. And serotonin levels are lowered when T3 levels become deficient—a more common occurrence than many doctors might suspect.[8]

Persistent, unrelenting stress will ultimately lead to adrenal exhaustion, poor stress coping abilities, and increased susceptibility to developing anxiety and depression. This stress includes the stimuli coming at us from TVs, radios, traffic, cell phones, pagers, electromagnetic pollution, and interpersonal interactions. Learn more about adrenal exhaustion in chapter 7.

An imbalance in essential fatty acids (EFAs) can also cause depression. EFAs are essential for our existence and cannot be manufactured by the body. They must be obtained from the foods we eat. Research shows that low blood levels of omega-3 EFAs, for instance, is linked to depression.[9]

In the next chapter I'll introduce you to my "Brain Function Questionnaire." This questionnaire will help you determine if you're deficient in one of the mood-regulating neurotransmitters. Once a deficiency is discovered, we can begin to correct it with the proper amino acid that will help your body to naturally heal itself by building the missing brain chemical. Let's get started!

1.*Linus Pauling in His Own Words,* Touchstone Books, New York, NY 1995.

2.Kunin, R.A., M.D. *Orthomolecular Psychiatry. In The Roots of Molecular Medicine: A tribute to Linus Pauling,* ed, R.P. Heumer, M.D. New York: W.H. Freeman and CO. 1986,180-213.

3.*JAMA,* September 14, 1994.

4.Roubenoff R, et al, "Malnutrition among hospitalized patients: problems of physician awareness." *Arch Intern Med* 147:1462- 1465.1987

5.Anderson RA, Poansky MM, Bryden NA, Canary JJ, "Chromium supplementation of humans with hypoglycemia." *Fed Proc* 43:471,1984.

6.Rogers SA, *Tired or Toxic?,* Prestige Printing, Box 3161, Syracuse NY 13220, 1990.

7.Russ C, Hendricks T, Chrisley B et al. "Vitamin B6 status of depressed and obsessive-compulsive patients." *Nutr Rep Intl* 1983;27:867-873

8.C.Kirkegaard and J. Faber, " The Role of Thyroid Hormone in Depression," *European Journal of Endocrinology* 138 (1998):1-9.

9.M.Maes et al., "Fatty acid composition in major depression: decreased omega-3 fraction in cholesteryl esters and increased C20:4 omega 6/C20:5 omega 3 ratio in cholesteryl esters and phospholipids," *Jour Affect Disord* 1996;38:35-46.

5

Interpreting the Brain Function Questionnaire

Before you begin this chapter,

complete the Brain Function Questionnaire in

Appendix A. Once you've determined which group(s)

your symptoms fall into, read on in *this* chapter.

THE "O" GROUP: OPIOIDS

The "O" Group is named for the **opioid neurotransmitters** contained in the hypothalamus gland. These neurotransmitters have two primary functions:

First, opioids are released in small bursts when we feel a sense of urgency (stress). Some individuals seem to feed off of this adrenaline rush. A sense of urgency can also help us get out of bed in the morning. However, if you can never turn this sense of urgency off, you'll eventually deplete the opioids, along with other vital hormones including cortisol and dehydroepiandrosterone (DHEA) hormone. Produced by the adrenal glands DHEA is a potent antidepressant in it's own right.

As a way to turn off the constant mind chatter, those in the "O" group use stimulants and mind-numbing chemicals (alcohol, marijuana, junk food, etc.) to escape the constant pressure they place on themselves to be more, do more, have more. These chemicals can temporarily relieve anxious feelings by providing artificial opioids. Unfortunately, these artificial opioids also cause the opioid-manufacturing cells in your brain to reduce output. These cells then lose their ability to produce the needed opioids, the body craves artificial opioids, and an addiction is born.

Second, when you exercise, your body releases extra opioids. This relieves sore muscles and may provide a feeling of euphoria. The opioids play an important role in pain modulation, so a deficiency of opioids can lower our pain threshold and make us more sensitive to painful stimuli.

SUPPLEMENT WITH PHENYLALANINE

DL-phenylalanine (a special form of the amino acid phenylalanine) can be extremely helpful in restoring proper opioid levels. Start with 1,000 mg. one–two times daily on an empty stomach (30 minutes before or one and a half hours after eating or taking another amino acid supplement). If you don't seem to notice any benefits, keep increasing the dose, up to 4,000 mg. twice a day (some of my patients are safely taking 6,000 mg. one–two times daily). If you experience rapid heartbeat, agitation, or hyperactivity, reduce or stop taking DL-phenylalanine. L-glutamine increases the effectiveness of DL-phenylalanine, so take 500 mg. of L-glutamine one–two times daily on an empty stomach.

Phenylalanine can increase blood pressure. If you already have high blood pressure, consult your doctor before taking any form of it. Phenylalanine can be stimulating and shouldn't be taken past 3:00 p.m. in the afternoon.

THE "G" GROUP: GABA

The "G" group symptoms are from the absence of the neurotransmitter **gamma-aminobutyric acid (GABA).** GABA is an important neurotransmitter involved in regulating moods and mental clarity. Tranquilizers used to treat anxiety and panic disorders work by increasing GABA. Instead of using a GABA additive loaded with side effects use an inexpensive $15 bottle of over-the-counter GABA. GABA is a great natural anti-anxiety supplement. It works rather quickly, within half an hour, doesn't cause fatigue or mental impairment and can be found at your local health food store.

GABA is made from the amino acid **glutamine.** Glutamine passes across the blood-brain barrier and helps provide the fuel needed for proper brain function. Once past the blood brain barrier, glutamine is able to turn into GABA.

A shortage of glutamine can reduce IQ levels, and glutamine supplementation has been shown to increase IQ levels in some mentally deficient children. That's because glutamine is brain fuel! It feeds the brain cells, allowing them to fire on all cylinders. A deficiency in glutamine can result in foggy thinking and fatigue. Individuals with mental fog, poor memory, or decreased mental acuity may benefit tremendously from supplementing this essential amino acid.

Even a small shortage of glutamine will produce unwarranted feelings of insecurity and anxiousness. Other symptoms include continual mental or physical fatigue, anxiety, depression, and occasionally, impotence.

SUPPLEMENT WITH GABA

Usually only a small dose of GABA is needed: 500–1,000 mg. twice daily. Some individuals may need to take it three–four times a day. Like most amino acids, GABA needs to be taken on an empty stomach, 30 minutes before or one and a half hour after eating. I've had considerable success using GABA with my anxiety patients.

OR USE THEONINE

I always start my anxiety patients on GABA first. However, some individuals may not notice much improvement from taking GABA or have unwanted side effects (burning in the stomach or flushing sensation). For these individuals I recommend a trial of the amino acid **L-theonine.** L-theonine is an amino acid found in green tea, and it has a calming effect on the brain. It easily crosses the blood brain barrier and increases the production of GABA. L-theonine also helps boost dopamine. Like GABA supplements, L-theonine doesn't cause drowsiness.

L-theonine as been shown to increase alpha waves, which are associated with meditative states of mind. Individuals taking L-theonine report feeling calm and relaxed. Research with human volunteers has demonstrated that L-theonine creates its relaxing effect in approximately 30 to 40 minutes after ingestion. The recommended dosage is 100–200 mg. taken as needed or 2–3 times a day on an empty stomach.

THE "D" GROUP: DOPAMINE

Dopamine is a neurotransmitter associated with the enjoyment of life: food, arts, nature, your family, friends, hobbies, and other pleasures. Cocaine's (and chocolate's) popularity stems from the fact that it causes very high levels of dopamine to be released in a sudden rush.

A dopamine deficiency can lead to a condition known as anhedonia— the lack of ability to feel any pleasure or remorse in life. It also reduces the person's attention span. The attention span of a person who has taken cocaine for some time is often reduced to two–three minutes, instead of the usual 50–60 minutes. Learning, for such a person, is nearly impossible. Brain fatigue, confusion, and lethargy are all by-products of low dopamine.

SUPPLEMENT WITH PHENYLALANINE

The brain cells that manufacture dopamine use the amino acid **L-phenylalanine** as raw material. Like most cells in the hypothalamus, they have the ability to produce four–five times their usual output if larger quantities of the raw materials are made available through nutritional supplementation. So the more L-phenylalanine the more dopamine.

Start with 1,000 mg. of L-phenylalanine one–two times daily on an empty stomach. If you don't seem to notice any benefits, keep increasing the dose, up to 4,000 mg. twice a day. If you experience a rare side effect like rapid heart-beat, agitation, or hyperactivity, reduce or stop taking L-phenylalanine. L-glutamine increases the effectiveness of L-phenylalanine, so take 500 mg. of L-glutamine one–two times daily on an empty stomach.

Phenylalanine can increase blood pressure. If you already have high blood pressure, consult your doctor before taking any form of it. Phenylalanine can be stimulating and shouldn't be taken past 3:00 in the afternoon.

THE "N" GROUP: NOREPINEPHRINE

The neurotransmitter **norepinephrine,** when released in the brain, causes feelings of arousal, energy, and drive. On the other hand, a short supply of it will cause feelings of a lack of ambition, drive, and/or energy. Deficiency can even cause depression, paranoia, and feelings of apathy.

Norepinephrine is also used to initiate the flow of adrenaline when you are under psychological stress. The production of norepinephrine in the hypothalamus is a 2-step process. The amino acid **L-phenylalanine** is first converted into tyrosine. Tyrosine is then converted into norepinephrine. Tyrosine, then, can be supplemented to increase norepinephrine (and dopamine). But too much tyrosine can cause headaches, so I usually recommend L-phenylalanine replacement first.

SUPPLEMENT WITH PHENYLALANINE

Start with 1,000 mg. of L-phenylalanine one–two times daily on an empty stomach. If you don't seem to notice any benefits, keep increasing the dose, up to 4,000 mg. twice daily. If you experience a rare side effect like rapid heartbeat, agitation, or hyperactivity, reduce or stop taking L-phenylalanine. L-glutamine increases the effectiveness of L-phenylalanine, so take 500 mg. of L-glutamine one–two times daily on an empty stomach.

Phenylalanine can increase blood pressure. If you already have high blood pressure, consult your doctor before taking any form of it. Phenylalanine can be stimulating and shouldn't be taken past 3:00 in the afternoon.

OR USE SAMe

An alternative to L-phenylalanine is **SAMe (S-adenosyl-methionine).** Pronounced "Sam-ee," it has been hailed as the safest and most effective natural antidepressant ever used. It is a molecule derived from the union of the amino acid methionine to a factor responsible for energy production, called adenosine triphosphate (ATP). SAMe increases the action of several neurotransmitters (dopamine, serotonin, and norepinephrine for example) by facilitating the binding of these hormones to their cell receptors.[1] It works rather quickly and seems to provide the needed pep that many of my patients are looking for.

SAMe also helps maintain mitochondrial function at peak levels, thus increasing energy production in the brain. In addition, SAMe has antioxidant properties, protecting brain tissues against damage from free radical damage. It also increases the production of the body's own glutathione, a strong antioxidant involved in many brain processes.[2]

There have been more than 100 peer-reviewed studies showing that SAMe is an effective, fast-acting, natural medication for depression,[3] and an analysis of the studies to date concluded that SAMe is *as effective as* any of the available prescription antidepressants on the market today.[4,5]

SAMe (along with serotonin) is also necessary for the synthesis of the sleep-regulating hormone melatonin. Elevated homocysteine levels block the production of SAMe leading to a melatonin deficiency and poor sleep. Homocysteine is a toxic chemical associated with heart disease, and increased levels may be a sign of depression.

I find that I'm recommending SAMe for my patients more and more often. And although studies show that some patients need up to 1200 mg. daily, my patients often don't need but 200–800 mg. when also taking the other core supplements I recommend. It may be that SAMe is able to work faster and perhaps better than L-phenylalanine to stabilize serotonin and epinephrine levels. I've had several patients comment that after they started SAMe, something "shifted," and they felt better— better than they had felt in a long time.

Not all SAMe is created equal, however. The price has come down for SAMe, but it is still around $30 for 30 200-mg. tablets. So you might be tempted to buy SAMe at a large discount store. Don't do it! SAMe starts to deteriorate rather quickly when exposed to air. It needs to be vacuum packed. I use SAMe that comes from directly from Italy. It has been used in Italian medicine for decades, and the SAMe from Italy is pharmaceutical grade and therefore the most effective. It's far superior to any other I've tried, and I believe that it's quality is why I'm getting such good results.

SAMe should be taken on an empty stomach. I recommend starting with 200–400 mg. of SAMe in the morning and, if needed, 200–400 mg. in the early afternoon. Some individuals may need to take up to 1200 mg. in divided doses. For most individuals, though, lower doses will be all they need to notice a change in their depression. SAMe can cause dry mouth and may increase blood pressure. It shouldn't be taken past 4 o'clock in the afternoon since its stimulating effects can interfere with your sleep.

THE "S" GROUP: SEROTONIN

Serotonin is a hypothalamus neurotransmitter necessary for sleep. A lack of serotonin causes difficulty in getting to sleep as well as staying asleep, and it is often this lack of sleep that causes the symptoms indicative of the "S" group.

Serotonin levels can easily be raised by supplementing with the essential amino acid **L-tryptophan,** but dietary supplements of L-tryptophan are banned in the US. However, **5-hydroxytryptophan (5HTP),** a form of tryptophan, is available over-the-counter and works extremely well for most patients.

SUPPLEMENT WITH 5HTP

If you fall into the "S" group, 5HTP might well change your life forever. When taken correctly, it turns right into serotonin. And serotonin will get instantly to work regulating your sleep, raising your pain threshold, and elevating your moods. Therapeutic administration of 5HTP has been shown to be effective in treating a wide range of health problems, including anxiety, depression, fibromyalgia, insomnia, binge eating, pain, and chronic headaches.

Studies (including double-blind experiments) comparing SSRIs and TCAs to 5HTP have consistently shown that 5HTP is *as good if not better than* these prescription medications at treating depression. And 5HTP doesn't have some of the more troubling side-effects.[6]

In one study evaluating the effects of 5HTP in individuals with uni- and bipolar depression, patients on 5HTP had a 50% reduction in their mood disorder symptoms.[7]

Consider these statistics from a study comparing 5HTP to the SSRI Luvox (fluvoxamine). The percentages indicate the patient's improvement on each type of treatment.[8]

Symptom	5HTP	Luvox
Anxiety	58.2%	48.3%
Depression	67.5%	61.8%

5HTP has also been show to help those who just aren't responding at all to prescription drug treatment. On average, 40% of patients will not respond to SSRI medications. Of these 40% who switch to older tricyclic drugs, 70% will respond. This still leaves a subgroup of patients who just aren't getting any help at all from prescription medications. Amazingly, administering 5HTP to these nonresponders helps 50% of them become depression free. This is a dramatic finding, since these nonresponders, on average, have been suffering from depression for about nine years! Drugs hadn't helped, but 5HTP did![9]

5HTP has been shown to be beneficial in treating insomnia, especially in improving sleep quality by increasing REM sleep (deep sleep). This is because 5HTP, with the help of certain vitamins and minerals, turns into serotonin and then into melatonin, a natural sleep hormone.[10] In fact, 5HTP can increase the body's production of melatonin by 200%.[11]

5HTP has been used to successfully treat and prevent chronic headaches including migraines, tension headaches, and juvenile headaches.[12]

Weight loss, if needed, can be a surprise benefit of 5HTP treatment. Clinical trials of obese individuals have demonstrated decreased food intake and subsequent weight loss with 5HTP supplementation.[13]

For my fibromyalgia patients, 5HTP is a first step on the road to wellness. One European study showed that the combination of MAOIs (such as Nardil or Parnate) with 5HTP significantly improved FMS symptoms, whereas other antidepressant treatments were not effective. The doctors conducting this study stated that a natural analgesic (pain blocking) effect occurred when serotonin and norepinephrine levels were enhanced in the brain. More norepinephrine means more energy and improved mood.[14]

A minority of people find that after being on 5HTP for several weeks or months, their improvement begins to decline. This is most likely due to an increased awareness of other neurotransmitter deficiencies (norepinephrine, GABA, dopamine, etc.). If this happens, I recommend adding 200–400 mg. of SAMe once or twice a day on an empty stomach (see dosing information above).

5HTP can also be beneficial in the treatment of IBS (irritable bowel syndrome). You might be surprised to know that you have more serotonin receptors in your intestinal tract than you do in your brain! (This is one reason people get butterflies in their stomach when they get nervous.) So low serotonin can certainly interfere with proper intestinal function. Symptoms associated with IBS (diarrhea and constipation) usually disappear within 1–2 weeks once serotonin levels are normalized.[15,16] And in my experience, once a person gets her serotonin levels up, IBS goes away, never to return. This is life-changing for many of my patients.*

If you're having problems falling asleep or staying asleep, begin with 50 mg. of 5HTP on an empty stomach 30 minutes before bed with four ounces of juice. The juice will cause you to release insulin, which helps 5HTP get past the blood-brain barrier and quickly boost brain serotonin levels.** If you still aren't sleeping well, increase your dose of 5HTP by 50 mg. each night (up to a maximum of 300 mg.) until you fall asleep within 30 minutes and stay asleep through the night. 5HTP will never make you feel dopey, drugged, or hungover, and it can be taken along with prescription sleep medications. A small percentage of those taking 5HTP at bedtime will actually become more alert. If this happens, simply stop taking 5HTP at bedtime. Take it instead with food during the day: 50 mg. with dinner for 1–2 days; if no problems, add up to 100 mg. at lunch and 200 mg. at dinner (up to 300 mg. daily).

Individuals in the "S" group who aren't having sleep problems should take about half of their 5HTP at a mealtime and the rest at bedtime.

I have a small percentage of patients who don't seem to notice much improvement at all from taking 5HTP. If this happens to you, add St. John's Wort to your 5HTP replacement therapy (if under the age of 50) or Ginkgo biloba (if age 50 or older).

---

*Please be aware that drugs often used to treat IBS can be very dangerous. These include smooth muscle relaxants (Bentyl, Levsin, and Levsinex), anti-diarrhea meds (Immodium, Lomotil), bulk-forming laxatives (Metamucil), and Zelnorm (a 5HT4 agonist). (5HT4 is not to be confused with 5HTP.) These medications range from innocuous to life endangering. Zelnorm's side effects include severe liver impairment, severe kidney impairment, bowel obstruction, diarrhea, constipation, abdominal pain, headaches, abdominal adhesions, gall-bladder disease, and back pain. Lotrinex (alosetron), a 5HT3 agonist, has been responsible for at least four deaths. Many who have taken the drug have reported severe abdominal pain from constipation. The drug was taken off the market but is now being approved with strict prescribing guidelines. An editorial in *The British Medical Journal* suggests that as many as 2 million Americans will be eligible for the drug under the new guidelines. According to previous reported side effects, this would result in 2,000 cases of severe constipation, almost 6,000 cases of ischemic colitis, 11,000 surgical interventions, and at least 324 deaths.

**Insulin-dependent diabetics should accompany the dose of 5HTP with the juice and a small bolus of insulin equal to treatment for one carbohydrate serving. Talk to your healthcare team to fit this safely into your meal plan.

FEELING OVERWHELMED?

You might have checked several statements in all the brain function categories. This is a sign that you're brain chemistry is in need of a major overhaul. Having more than one amino acid/neurotransmitter deficiency isn't uncommon. But before you start trying to figure out how you're going to take three different amino acid supplements, all on an empty stomach, let me help you get off to the right start.

1. Reduce stress. First of all, along with taking the recommended amino acids, I suggest you also start finding ways to reduce your stress. Clean up your diet; avoid sodas, caffeine, sugar, white flour, and processed foods, to help you body repair your brain chemistry. The chapters that follow go into more detail about ways to boost the effectiveness of the your amino-acid therapy by using the appropriate vitamins, minerals and essential fatty acids.

2. Boost brain function with vitamins and minerals. I recommend that everyone on amino-acid therapy take a high-potency optimal daily allowance multivitamin/mineral formula. *This is crucial!* I also recommend taking a minimum of 2,000 mg. of high-quality fish oil daily. Remember, you need plenty of certain vitamins and minerals, as well as essential fatty acids, to convert the amino-acids you're supplementing into the neurotransmitters that your brain is starving for.

3. Always start with 5HTP replacement therapy if you (1) checked three or more "S" group items or (2) are having trouble sleeping, even if you checked more statements in other areas. An example: if you checked five "O" group items, three "N" group items, and three "S" group items, begin by taking 5HTP for 1–2 weeks; then start adding DL-phenylalanine or SAMe. Here's another example: You checked five "N" group items and two "S" group items, but you're not having trouble sleeping. In that case, start the L-phenylalanine or SAMe as directed.

If you're having trouble falling to sleep or staying asleep, make *sure* you're taking 5HTP at bedtime. A good night's sleep is crucial to replenishing your stress-coping savings account.

FREQUENTLY ASKED QUESTIONS

Can I take 5HTP or some of the other amino acids if I'm taking anti-depressants or sleep medications?

Yes. Ninety percent of my patients are taking prescription antidepressant drugs. They don't make serotonin or epinephrine. Most antidepressants are like gasoline additives, they help a person hang on to the serotonin or epinephrine their brain is already producing. Most individuals don't have any serotonin or epinephrine in their brain to re-uptake. A gasoline additive doesn't help when the tank is empty! Most individuals with depression or mood disorders are deficient in serotonin and epinephrine; they've used it all up and their brains are empty. This is why they are depressed, have more pain, suffer from insomnia, and anxiety. Using a gasoline additive isn't going to help. Serotonin and epinephrine are made from the amino acids. Why use a gasoline additive (that has all kinds of potential side-effects) when you can just pour gasoline into your tank. Yes, please take amino acids along with your medications.

Should I stop taking my prescription medications?

I don't recommend you stop taking your prescription medications until after you start feeling better on my program. Stopping medications can trigger a host of withdrawal symptoms. Start taking the supplements I recommend, build your stress coping system up, and allow your body to start healing itself. After you start feeling stronger (it may be a few months) then with the help of your doctor, slowly start weaning off the medications. Most of the antidepressant medications can be weaned off and never missed. Some medications will have to be re-started until you become stronger or find other less toxic options. It's very important to work with your medical doctor when weaning off your prescription antidepressants or antianxiety drugs. I suggest taking 2–3 months to wean off these medications.

Remember you don't have to wait until you've weaned off your prescription drugs before beginning amino acid replacement therapy. Amino acids can be taken with prescription antidepressants and antianxiety drugs.

What if someone has a serotonin syndrome reaction?

Serotonin syndrome occurs when a person gets too much serotonin. This can cause rapid heartbeat, increased pulse rate, elevated blood pressure, agitation, and in its worst case scenario, irregular heartbeats (arrhythmia).

I have thousands of individuals on 5HTP and have seen only one person have a serotonin syndrome reaction. She was not a patient. She had a history of irregular heart beats and chemical sensitivities. She also had chronic fatigue syndrome. These individuals often have sluggish livers, which prevents them from efficiently processing supplements or medications. I would have never recommended she take 5HTP at bedtime. Instead, I would have had her start with 50 mg. with food (if I would have recommended it at all). She took 50 mg. at bedtime. The first night, it made her more alert (a sign not to take it at night). She then increased to 100 mg. the next night. She began having serotonin syndrome. This caused her to be anxious and have arrhythmia for the next few hours.

This is not to scare you. I use 5HTP (for sleep or depression disorders) with individuals with known heart conditions: including mitral valve prolapse and congestive heart failure. I always start with a low dose (50 mg.) and warn the patient to stop taking it at bedtime if she has a funny reaction. These people are on incredibly toxic heart medications that increase their risk for heart failure, stroke, and death. (For more information, see my book *Heart Disease: What Your Doctor Won't Tell You.*) If I don't get them to consistently go into deep restorative sleep each night, they'll never get well. So I don't worry about using 5HTP. Once you start reading about the medications and combinations of medications you've been taking, you'll know just how safe 5HTP is. I have been using 5HTP for the last 4–5 years and now have thousands of individuals taking it around the world.

What are some of the other potential side effects of 5HTP?

Other than some patients becoming more alert when taking 5HTP at bed time, I have very few complaints. The literature says that individuals may have headaches and nausea from taking 5HTP, but I have had less than half a dozen patients report this. The headaches and any nausea go away after a couple of days. Some patients will complain of fatigue when taking 5HTP during the day with food. If so, I have them take 100 mg. at lunch and 200 mg. at dinner. If they continue to have problems, I suggest they try 300 mg. at dinner.

See Appendix B for information on ordering recommended supplements.

1.Cohen BM, Stramentinoli G et al. "Effects of the novel antidepressant SAMe on alpha-I and beta adrenoceptors in rat brain." *Eur J Pharmacol,* 1989, 170(3):210-207.

2.De La Cruz JP et al. "Effects of chronic administration of SAMe on brain oxidative stress in rats." *NaunynSchmiedebergs Arch Pharmacol,* 2000, 361(l);47-52.

3.Mischoulon D, Fava M. "Role of 5-adenosyl-L-methionine in treatment of depression: a review of the evidence." *Am J Clin Nutr* 2002 Nov;76(5):11585–615.

4.Bressa, G,M. "S-Adenosyl-l-methionine (SAMe) as antidepressant: meta-analysis of clinical studies." *Acta Neurol. Scand. Suppl.* 1994; 154: 7-14.

5.Berlanga, C., Ortega-Soto, H.A., Ontiveros, M., Senties, H. "Efficacy of S-adenosyl-L-methionine in speeding the onset of action of imipramine." *Psychiatry Res.* 1992 Dec; 44(3): 257-62.

6.Birdsall T., "5-Hydroxytryptophhan: A Clinically Effective Serotonin Precursor" *Altern Med Rev* 1998;3(4):271-280.

7.Costa and Greengard (1984). "Frontiers in Biochemical Pharmacological Research in Depression." *Advances in Biochemical Psychopharmacology.* Vol 39, p. 301–13.

8.W. Poldinger, B. Calancini, W. Schwartz, "A functional-dimensional approach to depression: Serotonin defies=ciency as a target syndrome in comparison of 5HTP and fluvoxamine," *Psychopathology* 24 (1991): 53-81.

9.J.J. van Hiele, "L-5-hydroxytryptophan in depression: The first substitution therapy in psychiatry?" *Neuropsychobilogy* 6 (1980): 230-40.

10.Birdsall T., "5-Hydroxytryptophhan: A Clically Effective Serotonin Precursor" *Altern Med Rev* 1998;3(4):271-280.

11.ibid.

12.ibid.

13.ibid.

14.J. Angst, B. Woggon, and J. Schoepf, "The treatment of depression with L-5-hydroxytrptophan versus Imipramine: Results of two open and one double blind study," *Archiv fur Psychiatrie und Nervenkrankheiten* 224 (1997): 175-86.

15.Goldberg PA, Kamm MA, Setti-Carraro P, van der Sijp JR, Roth C. St. Mark's Hospital, London, UK. "Modification of visceral sensitivity and pain in irritable bowel syndrome by 5-HT3 antagonism (ondansetron)." *Digestion* 1996 Nov-Dec;57(6): 478–83

16.Delvaux MM. Gastroenterology Unit and Laboratory of Digestive Motility, CHU Rangueil, Toulouse, France. "Stress and visceral perception." *Can J Gastroenterol* 1999 Mar;13 Suppl A:32A–36A

6

A Good Night's Sleep

In epidemiological surveys of the general adult population, 14–20% of subjects with significant complaints of insomnia showed evidence of major depression; the rate of depression was less than 1% in those without sleep complaints.

Insomnia plagues one in three Americans, one-quarter of these complain of chronic insomnia. The National Commission on Sleep Disorder Research estimates that by the middle of the 21st century, over 100 million Americans will have difficulty falling asleep. And psychiatric disorders are the single largest cause of chronic insomnia in the sleep-clinic population.

Obviously, there is a link between depression/anxiety and poor sleep. In many cases, insomnia may be the only initial symptom in depressive mood disorder. Also, insomnia during major depression is a risk factor for suicide within one year of assessment. Besides psychiatric disorders, a large variety of clinical conditions such as arthritis, chronic fatigue syndrome, GI disorders, and cardio-respiratory conditions frequently cause insomnia. Certain abnormal sleep conditions, such as restless legs syndrome, are extremely prevalent in elderly; they frequently cause insomnia in this group. And sometimes, chronic insomnia (primary insomnia) can occur without any obvious physical or psychiatric illness.

Those with chronic insomnia often state that it affects every aspects of their lives. A poor night's sleep leads to a variety of daytime symptoms including irritability, change in mood, and reduced vigilance and alertness.[1]

These symptoms not only affect the quality of life but also result in billions of dollars in lost productivity. Sleep loss due to insomnia intensifies the pain associated with a medical disorder and may exacerbate associated medical and psychiatric disorders. Data from several longitudinal studies indicate that insomnia increases the risk of development of the first occurrence of psychiatric disorders, including major depression, anxiety disorders and substance abuse.[2]

THE TWO STAGES OF SLEEP

The first type of sleep is known as rapid eye movement or REM. During REM, the eyes, though closed, are rapidly moving back and forth. This is where dreaming takes place.

The second stage is called, simply enough, non-REM sleep; it is further divided into stages 1,2,3, and 4. Non-REM sleep is crucial for overall well being. Stages 1 and 2, while important in maintaining the correct sleep cycle, don't provide the restorative powers of stages 3 and 4.

Non-REM sleep begins soon after we start to fall asleep. The first two stages have a faster brain wave pattern (as measured by EEG) and are considered the lighter stages. As brain activity begins to slow, we enter into stages 3 and 4. This usually occurs one and a half hours after falling asleep. The non-REM cycle is then interrupted by ten minutes of REM sleep.

REM sleep elicits a flurry of brain activity. These cycles occur five–six times a night. The time spent in REM continues to lengthen and may last up to an hour in the final cycle of sleep. Consequently, if you're not dreaming, that's a sign that you're not going into deep sleep.

Many of my patients have been on so-called "sleep" medications that render them brain-numb for eight hours. Most of these powerful sedatives don't allow a person to go into deep restorative sleep. So the person has her eyes closed while she's knocked out for eight hours, but she doesn't receive the health benefits of deep restorative sleep. She will often feel hungover in the morning; rarely will she feel rested and refreshed. What a different experience from supplementing with natural, sleep-inducing supplements!

MELATONIN

The pineal gland is located at the base of our brain, and the ancient Greeks considered the pineal gland to be the seat of the soul. This thought may not be far off, since the pineal gland is responsible for releasing the hormone **melatonin.** Melatonin acts to regulate the body's circadian rhythm, especially the sleep/wake cycle. Very small amounts of melatonin are found in some meats, grains, fruits, and vegetables. It is also available as a dietary supplement, though it has no known nutritional value.

Melatonin is produced from the amino acid tryptophan, which turns into serotonin during the day but into melatonin at night. Your body has its own internal clock that helps regulate your natural cycle of sleeping and waking hours (or circadian rhythm) in part by controlling the production of melatonin. Normally, melatonin levels begin to rise in the mid- to late evening, remain high for most of the night, and then decline in the early morning hours. The retinas of the eyes are extremely sensitive to changes in light, and an increase in light striking the retina triggers a decrease in melatonin production—this is nature's wake-up call. Conversely, limited exposure to light increases melatonin production—nature's lullaby.

Natural melatonin levels decline gradually with age. Some older adults produce very small amounts of melatonin or none at all. Chronic episodes of stress can also lead to low levels of melatonin and so, poor sleep.

SEASONAL AFFECTIVE DISORDER

Since natural melatonin production is partly affected by a person's exposure to light, during the shorter days of winter, melatonin production may start earlier or, more often, later. This change can lead to symptoms of seasonal affective disorder (SAD), or winter depression.[3] One in 10 people, including children, suffer from SAD. Symptoms associated with SAD include depression, fatigue, lethargy, anxiety, and carbohydrate cravings.

One to two hours of exposure to bright, ultraviolet light will usually decrease melatonin levels to a normal level. Special ultraviolet (full spectrum) bright lights are found in various stores and catalogs, and individuals with SAD should use these lights every day during the winter months. Those suffering from insomnia should avoid bright lights two to three hours before bed.

Elements that can decrease melatonin levels include:
- exposure to bright lights at night
- exposure to electromagnetic fields such as digital clocks, TVs, radios, white-noise machines, electric blankets, window-unit air conditioners, or anything running on an alternating current (exposure to both static and pulsed magnetic fields has been shown to significantly decrease melatonin production in the pineal gland of experimental animals)
- NSAIDs, including Celebrex, Mobic, Aleve, Bextra
- SSRIs including Prozac, Zoloft, Celexa, Paxil, Lexapro
- anxiety meds (benzodiazepines) like Klonopin, Ativan, Xanax, Restoril
- anti-hypertensive meds (beta-blockers, adrenergics, and calcium channel blockers) including Inderal, Toprol, Tenormin, Lorpressor
- steroids
- over 3 mg. of vitamin B12 in a day.
- caffeine
- alcohol
- tobacco
- evening exercise (for up to three hours afterwards)
- depression

Some foods that contain melatonin include:
- oats
- sweet corn
- rice
- Japanese radish
- tomatoes
- barley
- bananas

Drugs that raise melatonin levels include:
- fluvoxamine (Luvox)
- desipramine (Norpramin)
- most MAOIs
- St. John's wort (acts like an MAOI)

SEROTONIN

Remember the stress-coping savings account I described? One of the best ways to make deposits into it is by entering deep restorative sleep. When a person goes into deep sleep, he makes more serotonin, and the more stress a person is under, the more serotonin he'll need.

Adequate levels of serotonin promote deep restorative sleep, which creates more serotonin. However, low serotonin creates poor sleep and further depletion of serotonin. Chronic pain, poor sleep, fatigue, mental fatigue, poor memory, irritable bowel syndrome, anxiety, and depression are common conditions associated with low serotonin states.

WHY NOT JUST TAKE AN ANTIDEPRESSANT?

To review the reasons why, let's revisit the analogy I shared in chapter 2. Antidepressant drugs have been used with varying degrees of success in treating the sleeplessness of anxiety and depression, and many of my patients are on SSRIS. These drugs are supposed to help a patient hang on to and use her naturally occurring stores of serotonin. But this treatment is like using a gasoline additive to help increase the efficiency of your car's fuel. Most of the patients I see are running on fumes; there is no gasoline in their tank (no serotonin in their brain)! A gasoline additive (SSRI) won't help.

And remember, most SSRIs also deplete melatonin levels; low melatonin leads to poor sleep; poor sleep leads to less serotonin; and less serotonin leads to depression!

WHAT ABOUT SLEEPING PILLS?

Short-term use of prescription sleeping pills can be helpful in restoring natural sleep rhythms. However, sleep medications aren't recommended for long-term use, and all have unwanted side effects. Each year, Americans consume 5 billion sleeping pills; 15,000 of these Americans die from sleeping pills.[4] Below is a sampling of common pills and their side effects.

• **Ambien** (zolpidem) is a short-acting drug that usually lasts for four–six hours. Some patients do well on Ambien; some build up a tolerance and need higher and higher doses until the medicine no longer works. Those with sluggish liver function should use this medication with caution. Common side effects include dizziness and diarrhea. Some patients complain of loss of coordination or concentration, amnesia (short-term memory loss), fatigue, headache, anxiety, and difficulty sleeping. Long-term use can result in back pain, flu-like symptoms, depression, constipation, upset stomach, joint pain, sore throat, urinary infection, and heart palpitations. Patients are cautioned against abruptly stopping the medicine, since withdrawal symptoms commonly occur.

- **Trazadone** (desyrel) is an antidepressant that increases serotonin levels, reduces anxiety, and promotes deep sleep. I've found this drug to be quite helpful when 5HTP or melatonin doesn't work. But it can cause early-morning hangover and common side effects include upset stomach, constipation, bad taste in the mouth, heartburn, diarrhea, rash, rapid heartbeat, mental confusion, hostility, swelling in the arms or legs, dizziness, nightmares, drowsiness, and fatigue.

- **Soma** (carisprodol) is a muscle relaxant that acts on the central nervous system. The most common complaint is its sedating nature. It can be helpful, especially if there is a great deal of muscle guarding or chronic unrelenting tightness. Side effects include fatigue, rapid heartbeat, dizziness, depression, breathing difficulties, chest tightness, and trembling. Soma doesn't allow deep sleep.

- **Elavil** (amitriptyline) is a tricyclic antidepressant that is very sedating. It can cause weight gain, early-morning hangover, neurally mediated hypotension (low blood pressure), depression, poor sleep, anxiety, and irregular heartbeat.

- **Flexeril** (cyclobenzaprine) is a muscle relaxant chemically similar to Elavil. Unlike many of the prescription medications for sleep, Flexeril does allow the patient to go into deep stage-4 (restorative) sleep. But it is quite sedating. It's side effects—including gastritis, drowsiness, dry mouth, nervousness (anxiety), dizziness, headache, fatigue, irritability, blurred vision, confusion, rapid heartbeat, low blood pressure, and a feeling of being hungover or "out of touch"—prevent most patients from remaining on this drug for very long.

- **Sonata** (zaleplon) is a hypnotic drug prescribed for sleep disorders. It is designed to last for only four hours; this supposedly helps prevent morning hangover. Side effects include drowsiness, fatigue, amnesia (memory loss, tingling or loss of feeling in hands and feet, out of touch with reality, fatigue, and depression.

- **Zanaflex** (tizanidine) is a muscle relaxant used for sleep disorders. Like other muscle relaxers, it can help with insomnia. But it doesn't produce deep, restorative sleep. It doesn't help increase serotonin levels; it only tranquilizes the nervous system. For this reason alone it should be avoided. Side effects include liver failure (at least three individuals have died from taking this medication), asthenia (weakness), somnolence (prolonged drowsiness or a trance-like condition that may continue for days), dizziness, UTI (urinary tract infection), constipation, liver injury, elevated liver enzymes, vomiting, speech disorder, blurred vision, nervousness (anxiety), hypotension, psychosis/hallucinations, bradycardia (slow heart action), pharyngitis (sore throat), and dykiensia (defect in voluntary movements). The stuff is poison!

THERE IS A BETTER WAY.

Instead of using gasoline additives (SSRIs) or potentially dangerous sleeping pills, I recommend you correct your low serotonin state by using 5HTP and if needed, melatonin.

Those suffering from anxiety or depression should use 5HTP instead of melatonin, even if they're having problems with their sleep. Remember the amino acid 5HTP turns into serotonin, and then into melatonin. Individuals suffering from anxiety and depression need to build up their serotonin stores. So start with replacing 5HTP first.

PROTOCOL FOR DEEP RESTORATIVE SLEEP

Take 5HTP on an empty stomach, 30 minutes before bed, with four ounces of juice. This allows it to get past the blood-brain barrier and be absorbed directly into the brain. (See page 47 for more specific information about dosing with 5HTP.)

5HTP will never leave you feeling dopey, drugged or hungover. If you need to wake up in the middle of the night to feed a baby or check on a sick child, you can, and then you should be able to go right back to sleep.

One of three things will happen when you start by taking 50 mg. of 5HTP at bedtime.

1. **You fall asleep** within 30 minutes and sleep through the night. If so, stay on this dose. If you start to have problems with sleep again, increase your dose of 5HTP as described in #2 below.

2. **It doesn't help.** This is a typical response to such a low dose. Continue to add 50 mg. each night (up to a max of 300 mg.) until you fall asleep within 30 minutes and sleep through the night. You should stay at the minimum dose needed for deep sleep (up to a maximum of at 300 mg. nightly).

3. You perk up. Instead of making you sleepy, the dose makes you more alert. This is due to a sluggish liver. Discontinue 5HTP at bedtime, and instead take 50 mg. with food for 1–2 days. Taking 5HTP with food will slow it down and allow the liver to process it like food. And taking 5HTP with food will not usually make you sleepy. If after 1–2 days, you have no further problems with 5HTP, increase your dose to 100 mg. with each meal (300 mg. a day). It might take a little longer to see positive results when taking 5HTP with food (1–2 weeks). But don't worry; you'll eventually build your serotonin stores up and start to see an improvement in your sleep, pain, moods, IBS, and energy.

QUESTIONS

What is the maximum amount of 5HTP that I can take?

Don't take more than 300 mg. in a day, though this whole dose can be taken at bedtime if needed. If you are taking your 5HTP with food throughout the day, however, you can take up to 400 mg. in 24 hours.

Can I take 5HTP along with sleep medications?

Yes. I don't recommend patients discontinue taking their sleep medications. Instead I suggest they start using 5HTP and increase the bedtime dose until they sleep through the night. At some point they should be able to work with their medical doctor and slowly wean off the prescription sleep medication. Remember all prescription sleep medications have side effects. I also remind my patients that 5HTP never causes a hangover, but a combination of 5HTP and prescription medication can.

What if I'm taking a prescription sleep medication and sleeping all night?

If you're taking a TCA or Trazadone, Ambien, or Flexeril, and you're falling asleep within 30 minutes, dreaming, and sleeping 7–8 hours, then you should continue taking the sleep medication. Add 5HTP (50 mg.) three times daily with food. If no problems arise after 2–3 days, increase to 100 mg. of 5HTP with each meal. Why take the 5HTP at all? Remember that the reason you're taking these prescription drugs is because you have a serotonin deficiency, not a drug deficiency. You want to build up your serotonin levels so that eventually you won't need prescription sleep medications.

What if I'm sleeping well while using a sleep medication that doesn't promote deep sleep?

Then you will definitely need to take 5HTP. Medications which don't promote deep restorative sleep include Zanaflex, Neurontin, Klonopin, Ativan, Xanax, Restoril, Dalmane, Doral, Halcion, Prosom, BuSpar, Librium, Serax, Tranxene, Valium, Risperdal, Symbyax, Topamax, and all muscles relaxants except Flexeril.

Try taking 5HTP along with these medications. If this combination makes you feel hungover the next day, try reducing the dose or frequency of your prescription medication *along with your medical doctor's consultation.* The medications can cause severe withdrawal symptoms if discontinued quickly.

Can 5HTP be taken with any *medications?*

Yes, 5HTP can be safely taken with all prescription medications. I wouldn't recommend 5HTP be used for patients with manic depression or schizophrenia. These conditions are best referred to an orthomolecular psychiatrist who specializes in these complicated disorders.

What if I still can't fall asleep and sleep through the night even when taking the maximum amount of 5HTP?

OK, nobody said this was going to be easy. Most people will be consistently sleeping through the night within a week of starting the 5HTP protocol. However, there are always those who won't. If after two weeks of taking the maximum dose of 5HTP the correct way, you are not falling asleep and staying asleep through the night, add melatonin supplementation to your routine.

Take 3 mg. of sublingual melatonin (which dissolves under your tongue for rapid absorption) 30 minutes before bed, along with the 300 mg. of 5HTP at bedtime.

What if I am taking the maximum amount of 5HTP, I can fall asleep within 30 minutes, but can't stay asleep?

Try taking 3 mg. of timed-release melatonin at bedtime.

Can I take 5HTP, melatonin, and *prescription sleep medications at the same time?*

Yes, but follow the advice above. Start with adding 5HTP to your sleep medication first. Only add melatonin later if truly needed.

I get sleepy after dinner but then catch my second wind right before bedtime, what should I do?

The problem is your cortisol levels, which are affected by stress and your body's circadian rhythm (sleep-wake cycle), are either too high or out of sync. Normally, cortisol secretions rise sharply in the morning, peaking at about 8 a.m. After its peak, cortisol production starts to taper off until it reaches a low point at around 1 a.m.

Fluctuations in cortisol levels can occur whenever normal circadian rhythms are altered by, for instance, travel through time zones (jet lag) or changes in work shifts. Even a new bedtime can drastically alter cortisol patterns, and these changes can lead to insomnia and poor sleep.

Some patients have trouble falling asleep because their cortisol levels are too high at bedtime. These are the individuals who get a little sleepy but then catch their second wind and can't fall asleep. They may be sleepy earlier in the evening but attempt to stay awake a little longer (they don't want to go to bed so early, or they want to finish with household chores, watching a movie, reading, etc). An adrenal cortex test profile would help uncover any abnormal cortisol fluctuations (see Appendix B for testing information).

This is why it is important to try to go to bed (preferably before 11:00 p.m.) and wake up at the same time each day. Establishing normal sleep and wake times is crucial in restoring normal circadian rhythms.

You can try supplementing with L-theonine along with phos-phatidylserine (PS). L-theonine boosts alpha brain waves and reduces mind chatter. PS is one of the key human brain phospholipids and is essential for normal neuron structure and function. Along with other essential fatty acids, it may also play a critical role in cognitive function, including maintaining concentration and memory. PS helps block the release of cortisol.[5]

To treat your problem, take 200–400 mg. of PS at dinner or two hours before bed, 100 mg. of L-theonine before dinner, and 100 mg. of

L-theonine one and half hours after dinner (on an empty stomach). Then use either your 5HTP or 5HTP-melatonin combination at bed time.

Also make sure you're taking a minimum of 500 mg. of magnesium a day. (This should be included in your optimal daily allowance multivitamin/mineral formula.)

What about blood sugar problems like hypoglycemia and diabetes? How do these affect treatment?

Some patients have bouts of hypoglycemia (low blood sugar) during the night, and this wakes them up, because low blood sugar stimulates the release of cortisol. If you're waking up during the night feeling shaky, eating half a banana or other carbohydrate-rich food should help you go back to sleep.

If your blood sugar tends to shoot up when you eat sweets or drink juices, try taking your 5HTP with water instead.

If you're a diabetic on insulin, accompany your dose of 5HTP with the juice *and* a small bolus of insulin equal to treatment for one carbohydrate serving. Talk to your healthcare team to fit this safely into your meal plan.

OTHER OPTIONS

Some of my patients have had success using natural herbal remedies. I've taken three of the best herbal remedies for sleep (Hops, Passion Flower leaf, and Chamomile flower) and combined them into one formula, which is available from our office. Order by phone or online, or look for it at your local health-food store.

If you've tried everything and feel like you're getting nowhere, consider ordering a Comprehensive Melatonin and an Adrenal Cortex Profile to find out why you can't get to or stay asleep at night (see Appendix B for ordering tests). I'd also recommend you consult your medical doctor for a trial of Trazadone, Ambien, Elavil, or Flexeril. Continue taking 5HTP along with the prescription medication. After a few months, and with your doctor's help, you may be able to wean off your prescription sleep medication and just use 5HTP and, if needed, melatonin.

For more information on ordering 5HTP, melatonin, or the Herbal Sleep Formula, please see Appendix B.

1.Phillips KD, Moneyham L, Murdaugh C, Boyd MR, Tavakoli A, Jackson K, Vyavaharkar M. "Sleep disturbance and depression as barriers to adherence." *Clin Nurs Res.* 2005 Aug;14(3):273-93.

2.Moo-Estrella J, Perez-Benitez H, Solis-Rodriguez F, Arankowsky-Sandoval G. "Evaluation of depressive symptoms and sleep alterations in college students." *Arch Med Res.* 2005 Jul-Aug;36(4):393-8.

3.Wehr T, et al. (2001). "A circadian signal of change of season in patients with seasonal affective disorder." *Archives of General Psychiatry,* 58(12): 1108–1114

4.Drs. Peter M. Brooks and Richard O. Day, *New Eng J of Med,* 1991;324(24): 1716–25.

5.Nerozzi, Dina et al, "Early Cortisol Escape Phenomenon Reversed by Phophatidyl Serine In Elderly Normal Subjects." *Clincal Trials Journal,* 1-89, vol 26 (1).

7

The Adrenals: Overworked and Underpaid

Just as we have a stress-coping savings account, we also have stress-coping glands responsible for monitoring and coordinating our responses to stress. The main stress-coping glands are known as the adrenals.

There is no escaping the fact that our society is suffering from the ill effects of stress. We live in a fast-paced society where good is never good enough, and more is always better.

Modern technology has allowed us to take our work with us no matter where we go. It is not uncommon to see a harried business executive "vacationing" by the pool and chatting voraciously into her cell phone or clicking the keyboard of her laptop. So much to do; so little time. Life and its demands seem to be increasing while our time for rest, relaxation, and play are decreasing.

Sixty hour work weeks, urban sprawl, traffic, pollution, eating on the run, and the never-ending demands of trying to keep up with the Joneses can all take its toll. It's easy to feel overwhelmed. And if you're not already feeling run down, anxious, or depressed, simply turn on the evening news to be reminded of just how tragic life can be.

How does your body respond to all this? Remember that our brains monitor and regulate our thoughts through electrochemical systems. These systems depend on having an adequate amount of chemicals to help us control our responses to stress. But chronic stress can lead to chemical deficiencies and mood disorders. In this way, psychosocial and environmental stressors are risk factors for depression. Research indicates that stressors in the form of social isolation or early-life deprivation may lead to permanent changes in brain function that increase susceptibility to mood disorders. Genetics studies have revealed that environmental stressors interact with depression-vulnerability genes to increase the risk of developing depression.[1]

I'm an avid runner; this is my escape. No cell phones, pagers, or quick text email allowed. I simply don't take these with me when I run. However, I've become accustomed to seeing my neighbors talking on the phone while they take their daily walk. They can't even enjoy the peace and quiet of being alone in nature. As I watch these stress-over-loaded people, I often think, *why not just have a coronary and get it over with?* It is no wonder that our society is witnessing the increased incidence of anxiety and depression. We simply don't know when to say, "Enough is enough! I need a break."

STRESS-BUSTERS: THE ADRENAL GLANDS

The adrenals are a pair of pea-sized glands located atop each kidney. Their main job is to monitor and respond to stress.

"Stress" can be any type of stimulus in the environment that knocks the body out of homeostasis, the body's innate system of balance. The "stress response" is a series of physiological adaptations that ultimately re-establishes this balance. The stress response primarily includes the secretion of two types of hormones from the adrenal glands: epinephrine (also known as adrenaline) and cortisol.

The adrenal gland is divided into two parts: the cortex and the medulla.

THE CORTEX

The cortex, the outer portion of the adrenal gland, produces the corticosteroids dehydroepiandrosterone (DHEA) and cortisol. Corticosteroids increase sodium retention and therefore blood pressure (that's why one sign of adrenal fatigue is hypotension). They also help to regulate blood sugar levels.*

- **DHEA** helps convert fatty acids, carbohydrates, and protein into energy. See more about this powerful hormone later in the chapter.

- **Cortisol,** since its discovery some 50 years ago, has gained increasing prominence in treatment of autoimmune diseases, allergies, asthma, and athletic injuries.

THE MEDULLA

The medulla is the smaller inner portion of the adrenal gland. When the body is under stress, the medulla produces epinephrine and norepinephrine.

- **Epinephrine** causes increased systolic blood pressure, pulse rate, and cardiac function. Its main function is to increase the rate and depth of respiration to allow more oxygen to reach the blood stream. (Epinephrine also inhibits the muscle tone of the stomach; that's why you may feel a "knot" in your stomach during times of stress.) The body also uses epinephrine to regulate circulatory, nervous, muscular, and respiratory systems during times of stress.

- **norepinephrine** increases both systolic and diastolic blood pressure. Norepinephrine is also an important neurotransmitter that helps increase mental and physical energy. And you already know that low norepinephrine levels are associated with depression. Abnormally elevated levels of norepinephrine also tend to cause anxiety.**

---

*Over the years, researchers have developed powerful synthetic forms of these steroids with stronger anti-inflammatory effects. The first synthetic corticosteroids were hailed as wonder drugs. Unfortunately in continued high doses, these corticosteroids cause adverse side effects which include depression, fluid retention, high blood pressure, bone loss, gastrointestinal ulcers, cataracts, and breathing disorders.

**Clearly, a *balance* in this essential brain chemical is needed. Individuals who tested high in the "G" group on the Brain Function Questionnaire suffer from severe anxiety or have manic depressive disorder and should *not* boost their norepinephrine levels. Individuals who tested high in the "N," "O," or "D" groups suffer from low norepinephrine levels and should be using the appropriate amino-acid therapy along with adrenal-restoring nutrients (see Appendix B for information on these nutrients).

ADRENAL EXHAUSTION

Stress reactions aren't just for emergencies anymore! People today experience stress reactions every few minutes, as they are bombarded by stimuli like honking horns, ringing phones, and (my favorite) computer crashes!

Persistent, unrelenting stress will ultimately lead to adrenal exhaustion. And once this exhaustion sets in, it's not long before the body begins to break down. Adrenal exhaustion is known to cause many of the same problems associated with other forms of poor health:[2]

- chronic headaches
- allergies
- nagging injuries
- low sex drive
- chronic infections
- cold hands and feet
- decreased sense of well-being (depression)
- hypoglycemia (low blood sugar)
- hypotension (low blood pressure)
- neurally mediated hypotension (becoming dizzy or even fainting when standing up)
- fatigue
- decreased mental acuity
- low body temperature
- decreased metabolism
- a compromised immune system
- unhealthy weight loss
- hyperpigmentation (excess skin color changes)
- loss of scalp hair
- excess facial or body hair
- vitiligo (changes in skin color)
- auricular calcification (calcium deposits in the earlobe)
- GI disturbances
- nausea
- vomiting
- constipation
- abdominal pain
- diarrhea
- salt cravings
- muscle and joint pains

GENERAL ADAPTATION SYNDROME

The general adaptation syndrome (GAS) is our body's path to adrenal exhaustion. It is divided into three phases.

1. **Fight or flight:** This first phase is an alarm reaction triggered by messages in the brain that cause the pituitary gland to release adreno-corticotropic hormone (ACTH). This hormone then causes the adrenal glands to secrete adrenaline, cortisol and other stress hormones. The fight-or-flight response encourages the body to go on red alert and be ready for physical and mental activity. The heart beats faster to provide blood to the muscles and brain, and the breath rate increases to supply extra oxygen to the muscles, heart, and brain. Digestion and other functions not essential for maintaining the alarm reaction are halted. The liver rids itself of stored glycogen and releases glucose into the blood stream. The body is now ready for any real or imagined danger.

2. **Resistance:** While the alarm reaction is usually short-lived, the resistance reaction can last for quite some time. The major player in this phase is the hormone cortisol, secreted by the adrenal glands. Cortisol helps increase cellular energy and acts as a potent anti-inflammatory. It can be a lifesaver when used in allergic reactions (such as anaphylactic shock). Through cortisol, the resistance reaction allows the body to endure ongoing stress (such as pain, fatigue, or injury) for long periods of time. However, long-term stress can generate a host of health problems including high blood pressure, anxiety, fatigue, headaches, hypoglycemia, decreased immune function, thyroid dysfunction, diabetes, and adrenal exhaustion.

3. **Exhaustion:** This third stage is a result of chronic oversecretion of cortisol, and it accelerates the downward spiral towards chronic poor health.

Many of my patients suffering with mood disorders are also suffering from adrenal exhaustion. They have literally burned out their stress-monitoring organ.

THE IMPORTANCE OF DHEA

The adrenal cortex, when healthy, produces adequate levels of DHEA, which boosts our energy, sex drive, resistance to stress, self-defense mechanisms (immune system), and general well-being. But chronic stress causes the adrenals to release extra DHEA, and eventually they simply can't produce enough

DHEA serves as a parent compound for estrogen and testosterone, which have both been shown to enhance mood. DHEA is extremely important for normal brain function and helps prevent the destruction of tryptophan (5HTP), which increases the production of serotonin. In this way, DHEA provides added protection from chronic stress. Studies continue to show low DHEA to be a biological indicator of stress, aging, and age-related diseases including neurosis, depression, peptic ulcer, IBS, and others.[3]

The brain is the largest user of DHEA. It contains six and a half times more DHEA than any other organ. Our DHEA levels steadily rise beginning with puberty, peaking at about the age of 25. By age 70 or 80, DHEA levels have usually fallen to 10% of their peak values. Research shows that DHEA replacement therapy is helpful in treating adrenal insufficiency and in improving well-being in menopausal women and elderly men.[4,5]

DHEA has also been shown to be a potent antidepressant, countering elevated levels of cortisol associated with mania and anxiety disorder. Women with the least DHEA are the most likely to be depressed. And the lower the DHEA level, the more depressed the person becomes. Interestingly, levels of DHEA in one study correlated with mood even within the normal range.[6,7,8] DHEA also has anti-stress effects that may be part of its antidepressant action.

Studies have demonstrated that DHEA helps promote feelings of calmness. People who practice transcendental meditation have higher levels of DHEA than those who don't, and people who took part in a stress-reduction program were able to increase their DHEA by 100%. At the same time, they reduced their stress hormone levels by 23%.[9]

DHEA BOOSTS...

- energy
- sex drive
- resistance to stress
- immunity
- general well-being

AND HELPS TO RAISE...

- cortisol levels
- overall adrenal function
- mood, acts as an antidepressant
- cellular energy
- mental acuity
- muscle strength
- stamina[10]

SELF- TESTS FOR ADRENAL FATIGUE

I recommend that you do one of the following tests to see if you're suffering from adrenal fatigue:

- **Ragland's sign** is an abnormal drop in blood pressure when a person arises from a lying to a standing position. There should be a rise of 8–10 mm. in the systolic (top) number when you stand up. A drop in blood pressure—or failure to rise—indicates adrenal fatigue. Example: Someone takes your blood pressure while you're lying on your back. The systolic number is 120 and the diastolic number is 60 (120 over 60). Then blood pressure is taken again immediately after you stand up. The systolic number (120) should go up 10 points (from 120 to 130). If it doesn't increase 10 points, this indicates adrenal fatigue.It's not unusual for the systolic number to actually drop 10 or more points in my patients; this is a *sure* sign of adrenal fatigue.

- **Pupil dilation testing** is an easy test for adrenal dysfunction that you can do yourself with a flashlight and a mirror. Simply face the mirror, and shine the light in one eye. If after 30 seconds the pupil (black center) starts to dilate (enlarge), adrenal deficiency should be suspected. Why does this happen? During adrenal insufficiency, there is a deficiency of sodium and an abundance of potassium, and this imbalance causes an inhibition of the sphincter muscles of the eye. These muscles would normally initiate pupil constriction in the presence of bright light. However, in adrenal fatigue, the pupils actually dilate when exposed to light.

TESTING AND TREATING DHEA LEVELS

It is best to work with your doctor and have your DHEA levels checked before beginning supplementation. I use saliva adrenal hormone profiles to test for adrenal and DHEA deficiencies. For information on ordering this test, please see Appendix B.

Although I recommend everyone be tested for DHEA level, I sometimes begin patients on a low dose (5–25 mg. for females and 50 mg. for males) of DHEA based on symptoms. I believe DHEA replacement therapy to be relatively safe, even without testing. However, too much DHEA *can* cause side effects in those who aren't suffering from a deficiency. Females may experience facial hair growth (though I've seen this rarely in my 10 years of using DHEA, and then only from doses exceeding 100 mg.) or increased estrogen/progesterone levels. Men may experience symptoms associated with elevated testosterone, such as aggression, anxiety, and irritability.

While these are certainly unwanted side effects, I've found them to be rare and worth the risks. Most of the patients I treat for anxiety and depression are severely low in DHEA and have several symptoms of low DHEA which are much worse than the possible side effects. DHEA replacement therapy can often yield dramatic results in some of my more bewildering cases.

IMPORTANT CAUTIONS

Elevated cortisol or epinephrine levels can cause anxiety. Individuals with high anxiety levels or who suffer from manic-depression should *not* try to boost these unless working along with a knowledgeable doctor.

If you checked four or more "G" items on the Brain Function Questionnaire, please use 5HTP, GABA, and/or L-theonine along with essential fatty acids (discussed in chapter 10), and a good comprehensive multivitamin/mineral formula for a few months *before* starting any adrenal-restoring supplements (other than DHEA, which has a calming effect on the body).

ADRENAL RESTORATION PROTOCOL

Once you have determined that your adrenal glands are exhausted, you can get started helping heal them by following the steps below.

1. Use the appropriate amino acid replacement therapy as outlined in chapter 5.

2. Jealously guard your sleep, and make sure that it is consistently deep and restorative. See chapter 6.

3. Take a comprehensive optimal daily allowance multivitamin and mineral formula daily. See chapter 9.

4. Take DHEA if indicated on your saliva adrenal hormone profile. I've found sublingual (dissolving under the tongue) to be the best form of DHEA, but micronized forms of DHEA are also a good choice.

5. Consider taking adrenal cortical extracts. These supplements do contain DHEA and cortisol, however, so if you're concerned about anxiety-related problems, avoid these products and just stick with DHEA.

Adrenal cortical glandular extracts help repair and restore normal adrenal function: "Adrenal extracts have been recommended and successfully used for a variety of conditions that involve low adrenal function, including asthenia, asthma, colds, burns, depletion from infectious diseases, from colds, coughs, dyspepsia (poor digestion) early Addison's disease, hypotension (low blood pressure), infections, infectious diseases…neurasthenia (low energy/weakness), tuberculosis, light-headedness and dizziness, and vomiting during pregnancy."[11]

Adrenal extracts are not a new treatment. In the 1930s, they were very popular, used by tens of thousands of physicians. They were still being produced by leading drug companies as recently as 1968. Today, these extracts are available without a prescription as adrenal cortical glandular supplements.

Adrenal cortical extracts are still used to replenish and eventually normalize adrenal function. They have an advantage over prescription cortisol hormone replacement in that they can be instantly discontinued once they have done their job of repairing adrenal function. Adrenal extracts can also increase energy and speed recovery from illness.

I recommend starting with 500 mg. of adrenal cortex glandular twice a day with food. You should see a difference on the orthostatic blood pressure test and/or the pupil test within one to two weeks. If these tests don't improve within two weeks, double the dose of adrenal cortex, and retest in another two weeks.

Important: *Don't* use "whole gland adrenal" or "adrenal medulla glandular." These are designed to increase adrenaline levels and can cause anxiety, rapid heartbeat, and elevated blood pressure. I used whole adrenal glandular early on but found that some of my patients were having trouble with rapid heart rate, upset stomach, and high blood pressure when taking these supplements. Use only *adrenal cortex glandular* supplements.

6. Increase your vitamin-C intake; it's perhaps the most important nutrient in facilitating adrenal function and repair. Dr. James Wilson, author of *Adrenal Fatigue: The 21st-Century Stress Syndrome,* writes that "The more cortisol made, the more vitamin C is used. Vitamin C is so essential to the adrenal hormone cascade and the manufacture of adrenal steroid hormones that before the measurement of adrenal steroid hormones became available, the blood level of vitamin C was used as the best indicator of adrenal function level in animal research studies."[12] I recommend all patients take a minimum of 1,000–2,000 mg. daily of vitamin C.

7. Start an exercise program. Exercise may be one of the best ways to reduce stress and beat the ill effects of depression. Several studies have shown that exercise significantly reduces depressive symptoms.[13]

Walking has been shown to increase the efficient use of serotonin in the brain. From Dr. F. Batmanghelidj, MD, and his book *Your Body's Many Cries for Water* comes this quote: "There is a direct relationship between walking and the buildup of the brain's Tryptophan reserves." Dr. Batmanghelidj goes on to write about tryptophan's importance: "The brain Tryptophan content, and its dependent neurotransmitter systems, are responsible for maintenance of the 'homeostatic balance of the body.' Normal levels of Tryptophan in the brain maintain a well-regulated balance in all functions of the body—what is meant by homeostasis. With a decrease in Tryptophan supply to the brain, there is a proportionate decrease in the efficiency of all functions in the body."[14]

I don't recommend you begin a strenuous exercise program out of the blue. Even walking should be done with restraint until you become stronger and feel better on the supplements I recommend in this book. Exercise is a stress. A good stress, but a stress never the less. Until you build up your stress-coping savings account and are consistently sleeping through the night, I wouldn't recommend any exercise beyond walking for 10–20 minutes a day. Once you feel stronger, increase your walking to up to an hour a day. Don't push it; start slow and gradually increase over time.

Researchers from Duke University Medical Center found that exercise was just as beneficial as the SSRI medication Zoloft in reducing the symptoms associated with depression. The researchers divided 156 depressed men and women into three treatment groups: aerobic exercise (using a treadmill or stationary bicycle for 30 minutes, 3 times a week); Zoloft medication; and combined exercise and medication. Initially, people who took Zoloft improved faster, but after 16 weeks of treatment, all three groups experienced similar benefits. Six months after the trial ended, the benefits of exercise endured. In fact, individuals from the exercise-only group had significantly lower relapse rates than either those in the Zoloft-only or Zoloft-plus-exercise groups.[15,16]

8. Eat breakfast, and never skip meals. Individuals with low adrenal function are usually not hungry when they wake up. Healthy cortisol levels are at their highest around 8:00 a.m., and in an attempt to keep otherwise low cortisol levels elevated in the morning, people may prefer not to eat breakfast. They instead rely on chemical stimulants (coffee, sodas, cigarettes, etc.) to get them going. These stimulants temporarily raise blood sugar levels as well as serotonin levels. They also increase adrenaline and cortisol levels, which curbs the appetite even further.

But every artificially induced high is always followed by a self-correcting low. These low blood-sugar states often trigger feelings of anxiousness, mental fatigue, fuzzy thinking, and depression. The body needs a continuos supply of healthy non-stimulating nutrients throughout the day.

In addition, low adrenal function can make you to feel nauseated, so eating is the last thing you want to do. Eat breakfast anyway! A small healthy snack is all you need until hunger comes, usually a couple of hours later. Then eat another balanced snack to tie you over until lunch. Then, don't skip lunch!

The brain especially needs to fed; 40% of all foodstuff fuel goes to maintain proper brain function. So skipping meals can cause serious problems, especially with already established mood disorders.

9. Slowly reduce caffeine consumption. I'm betting that you're addicted to something to some extent: caffeine, nicotine, sugar, alcohol. You *must* work to eliminate—or at least limit—these adrenal-hormone robbers. I know this can be tough. But if you want to get well, this is really not an option. Remember to reduce all caffeine consumption, including caffeinated teas (green tea is fine), coffees, and sodas. Don't forget chocolate! The less caffeine, the better.

To prevent withdrawal symptoms (headaches, mood disturbances, fatigue), wean off caffeine over two–four weeks. Start by eliminating one quarter of your daily caffeine consumption. Consider each cup of caffeinated coffee, soda, diet soda, or tea, and each chocolate bar as one caffeine serving. If you consume four cups of coffee in the morning, three glasses of tea at lunch, and a diet Coke at dinner, consider this eight servings of caffeine for that day. Reduce your caffeine servings by one quarter (two servings). This would still allow you six servings a day. After seven days, reduce your caffeine servings by another quarter (in this case, 1.5 servings). Wait another five days, and then reduce the daily caffeine servings by half. Slowly discontinue all caffeine consumption over a manageable period of time.

10. Monitor your blood sugars to combat hypoglycemia. You don't have to be diabetic to have a problem with your blood sugars. And you can tell a lot about your blood sugars just by listening to your body. Alternatively, you can easily check your blood sugars with an at-home glucometer; ask your medical doctor for a prescription.

Avoid simple sugars. As any "sugarholic" can attest, a soda, doughnut, or pastry can provide a quick energy fix. But this rise in blood sugar is followed by a nosedive. And low blood sugar produces all the unwanted symptoms associated with mood disorders: fatigue, irritability, anxiety, mental fog, depression, and more.

To avoid the ups and downs of blood sugar swings, eat a balanced diet of whole, unprocessed foods. Some individuals will find they feel better eating several small or light meals spaced throughout the day.

Hypoglycemia (low blood sugar) is a complex set of symptoms caused by faulty carbohydrate metabolism. If you suffer from it consistently, you probably know that *something* is wrong. Hypoglycemia can make you feel terrible. One sure sign is sugar cravings, as you body calls out for a quick fix for what it needs. Normally, the body maintains blood sugar levels within a narrow range through the coordinated effort of several glands and their hormones. But if these hormones, especially glucagon (from glucose) and insulin (produced in the pancreas), are thrown out of balance, hypoglycemia or type-2 diabetes can result.

Hypoglycemia (in people not taking insulin) is usually the result of consuming too many simple carbohydrates (sugars). "Syndrome X" describes a cluster of abnormalities that owe their existence largely to a high intake of refined carbohydrates leading to the development of hypoglycemia, excessive insulin secretion, and glucose intolerance. This condition is followed by decreased insulin sensitivity, elevated cholesterol levels, obesity, high blood pressure, and type-2 diabetes.

Numerous studies have demonstrated that depressed individuals have faulty glucose/insulin regulatory mechanisms. Other studies have clearly shown the relationship between low blood sugar and decreased mental acuity.

The following foods are not recommended for anyone with hypoglycemia or hypoadrenia tendencies: table sugar, maltose, honey, sucrose (fruit sugar), bananas, raisins, dates, fruit juices, apricots, beets, white flour, white potatoes, white rice, cooked corn, corn flakes, and cereals.

In addition, individuals suffering from hypoglycemia should avoid all food listed high on the "glycemic index." The glycemic index is a measurement of how much a carbohydrate elevates the eater's circulating blood sugar. The lower the glycemic index, the slower the rate of absorption. Here's a sample list of foods and their glycemic index:

High Index	Moderate Index	Low Index
white bread	sourdough bread	pumpernickel bread
white potatoes	most pasta	most fruits
simple sugars	wild rice	meat and fish
white rice	brown rice	cheese
sweets	some beans	most vegetables

You can find out the glycemic index of just about any food that you can imagine by visiting the "GI Database" at www.glycemicindex.com.

It's best to combine protein, fat, and carbohydrate in each snack or meal. Avoiding simple sugars and consuming a balanced diet helps stabilize blood sugar levels. Eating healthy snacks throughout the day can also help keep your blood sugar levels stable. One simple snack that combines protein, fat, and carbohydrate is a handful of nuts (such as cashews, almonds, walnuts, or pecans) along with an apple, pear, or whole wheat crackers.

11. Combat hypoglycemia with supplements if needed. If you're following my adrenal restoration protocol, you'll probably not need any of the following supplements. However, some individuals with severe hypoglycemia can benefit from them.

• **Chromium** is a trace mineral that helps reduce glucose-induced insulin secretion. It works with insulin to facilitate the uptake of glucose into the cells. Glucose levels remain elevated in the absence of chromium. A normal dose is 200 mcg. Taken 30 minutes before or after meals, two–three times daily.

- **Vitamin B3** (niacin) helps regulate blood sugar levels and may help alleviate the symptoms of hypoglycemia. This should be in your multivitamin and mineral formula.

- **Magnesium** levels must be sufficient in order to avoid hypoglycemic reactions. This should be in your multivitamin and mineral formula.

- **Zinc** levels must be sufficient in order to avoid hypoglycemic reactions. This should be in your multivitamin and mineral formula.

- **L-glutamine,** an amino acid discussed earlier, helps regulate blood sugar levels. I've found it to be very effective in eliminating sugar cravings and hypoglycemic episodes. A normal dose is 500–1,000 mg. once or twice daily on an empty stomach.

- **Gymnema sylvester** is a climbing plant found in Asia and Africa. It's used in Ayruvedic medicine, an indigenous healing practice from India, for the treatment of type-2 diabetes. Scientific studies have shown this herb to be a valuable addition in preventing the symptoms of hypoglycemia. It's also routinely used to reduce sugar cravings.

In this chapter we've looked the effects of stress and adrenal fatigue. In the next chapter we'll take a look at how chronic stress, low adrenal function, and low thyroid are related. Low thyroid has been linked to mood disorders.

For information on ordering adrenal cortex glandular supplements, DHEA, or adrenal cortex stress profile saliva test kits, please see Appendix B.

1.Howard Z. Lorber, CSW, from NIH Publication NO. 00-4501 MAY 2000,

2.List composed from personal experience and from *Safe Uses of Cortisol* by William Jefferies, MD, FACP. Charles C. Thomas Publisher , LTD 1996 Springfield IL

3.Vermeulen A. "Adrenal androgens and aging." In: Genazzani AR, Thijssen JH, Siiteri, PK, editors. *Adrenal androgens.* New York: Raven Pres, 1980: 27–42.

4.Yen, S.S. et al. "Replacement of DHEA in aging men and women. Potential remedial effects." *Ann. N.Y. Acad. Sci.* 1995 Dec 29; 774: 128-42.

5.Morales, A.J. et al. "The effect of six months treatment with a 100 mg daily dose of dehydroepiandrosterone (DHEA) on circulating sex steroids, body composition and muscle strength in age-advanced men and women." *Clin. Endocrinol.* 1998 Oct; 49(4): 421-32.

6.Wolkowitz, O.M. et al. "Double-blind treatment of major depression with dehydroepiandrosterone." *Am. J. Psychiatry* 1999 Apr; 156(4): 646-9.

7.Bloch, M. et al. "Dehydroepiandrosterone treatment of midlife dysthymia." *Biol. Psychiatry* 1999; 45: 1533-41.

8.Barrett-Connor, E., von Muhlen, D., Laughlin, G.A., Kripke, A. "Endogenous levels of dehydroepiandrosterone sulfate, but not other sex hormones, are associated with depressed mood in older women: the Rancho Bernardo Study." *J. Am. Geriatr. Soc.* 1999 Jun; 47(6): 685-91.

9.Glaser, J.L. et al. "Elevated serum dehydroepiandrosterone sulfate levels in practitioners of the (TM) and TM-Sidhi programs." *J. Behav. Med.* 1992 Aug; 15(4): 327-41.

10.*Textbook on Physiology* by Guyton

11. *Applied Kinesiology: the Advanced Approach in Chiropractic* by David Walther, 1976

12.*Adrenal Fatigue The 21st Century Stress Syndrome,* by James L. Wilson, ND, DC, PhD. Smart Publications 2002

13.Paluska, S.A., Schwenk, T.L. "Physical activity and mental health: current concepts." *Sports Med.* 2000 Mar; 29(3): 167-80.

14.Global Health Solutions, 1992

15.Blumenthal, J.A., Babyak, M.A. et al. "Effects of exercise training on older patients with major depression." *Arch. Intern. Med.* 1999 Oct 25; 159: 2349-56.

16.Babyak, M., Blumenthal, J.A. et al. "Exercise treatment for major depression: maintenance of therapeutic benefit at 10 months." *Psychosom. Med.* 2000 Sep-Oct; 62: 633-8.

8

Thyroid Dysfunction

Over 20 million Americans suffer from thyroid
dysfunction, and more than 10 million women have a
low-grade thyroid dysfunction. Over 500,000 new
cases of thyroid disease occur each year.[1]

When your thyroid gland produces too much thyroid hormone, this is known as hyperthyroid. When your thyroid doesn't produce enough thyroid hormone, it's called hypothyroid.

The thyroid gland is shaped like a butterfly and is located in the lower front part of your neck (just above the breastbone). This gland is responsible for secreting thyroid hormones, which travel through the bloodstream and help cells convert oxygen and calories to energy. Basically, thyroid hormones control a person's metabolism.

Metabolism is defined as the sum of all physical and chemical changes that take place within the body; it's all the energy and material transformations that occur within living cells. Every cell in the body depends on having enough thyroid hormone, so if your thyroid gland becomes dysfunctional, every cell in the body suffers. This is why thyroid disorders can cause so many problems. On the next page are some symptoms associated with Hypothyroid[2]

- fatigue (the most profound symptom)
- depression
- headache
- dry skin
- swelling
- weight gain
- cold hands and feet
- poor memory
- hair loss
- hoarseness
- nervousness
- joint and muscle pain
- burning or tingling sensations in the hands and/or feet (hypothyroid neuropathy)
- yellowing of skin from a build up of carotene (conversion of carotene to vitamin is slowed by hypothyroidism)
- carpal tunnel syndrome
- problems with balance and equilibrium (unsteadiness or lack of coordination)
- constipation (from slowed metabolism)
- myxedema (nonpitting edema due to the deposition of mucin in the skin) around the ankles, below the eyes, and elsewhere
- observation of delayed Achilles tendon reflex test
- hypertension
- angina
- atherosclerosis
- hypercholesterolemia
- hyperhomocysteinemia
- menstrual irregularities
- infertility
- PMS
- fibrocystic breast disease
- polycystic ovary syndrome
- reactive hypoglycemia
- psoriasis
- urticaria
- vasomotor rhinitis
- allergic rhinitis

Statistics show that as many as 10 million Americans suffer from borderline hypothyroidism.[3] Some experts have suggested that hypothyroid disorders are woefully underreported and estimate that tens of millions of individuals with low thyroid go undiagnosed.

UNDERSTANDING THYROID HORMONES

The hypothalamus stimulates the pituitary gland (both are contained in the brain) to produce thyroid-stimulating hormone (TSH). TSH then stimulates the thyroid gland to produce and release the hormone thyroxine (T4). T4 hormone is then converted into triiodthyronine (T3). T3 hormone is essential for life and four times more active than T4. You can live without T4 but not without T3. A thyroid gland that functions normally produces both of them. Twenty percent of the T3 circulating in the body comes directly from the thyroid gland, and the remaining 80% comes from conversion of T4.

This conversion of T4 to T3 takes place in the cells. (T4 can also be converted into reverse T3 (rT3), which is physiologically inactive.)

The enzyme 5-deiodinase converts T4 into T3 and rT3. This enzyme can be inhibited by prolonged stress, acute and chronic illness, steroids (such as cortisol), and poor nutrition.

SHORTFALLS OF BLOOD TESTING

Blood tests for thyroid function measure the amount of TSH, T4, and T3 in the bloodstream. But thyroid hormones don't operate within the bloodstream; the action takes place in the cells themselves. What good is a blood test that only shows what is racing around the bloodstream one second out of one minute, out of one hour, out of a one day? Blood tests are an educated guess based on the bell curve theory. Sixty percent of patients will have thyroid levels between the usual testing parameters; 20% will be above; and 20% will fall below these parameters.

When I arrive at my office each morning, I can make an educated guess about the number of patients I have scheduled for that first hour. If there are 10 cars in the parking lot, my waiting room is probably full. However, I'm only guessing. Some of the car owners may be in the pediatric clinic next door. And even though six out of ten times, if there are 10 cars in the parking lot, six of those carloads will be in my waiting room and the rest in the pediatric clinic, all it takes is the a bad outbreak of flu and all 10 of the carloads are in the pediatric clinic (while my patients have had to park elsewhere). This is the kind of educated guess that doctors have to make when they rely on blood test results to evaluate thyroid function.

The *Journal of Clinical Psychiatry* has reported that "Laboratory blood tests for thyroid may be inaccurate for many who get tested for hypothyroid disorder."[4]

Compounding the problem of using standard blood tests to diagnose hypothyroid is the inability of doctors to agree on laboratory parameters for interpretation.

According to the American Association of Clinical Endocrinologists (AACE) guidelines, doctors have typically been basing their diagnoses on the "normal" range for the TSH test. The range of normal TSH levels, at most laboratories, has traditionally been 0.5–5.0. Those with a TSH below .5 are considered to have too much thyroid hormone (hyperthyroid), and those whose test results are above 5 are considered to have too little thyroid (hypothyroid). However, it's not uncommon to find doctors, including endocrinologists, who withhold the diagnosis and treatment of hypothyroid until a patient's TSH tests register considerably above 5. Conversely, some doctors believe that anyone with a TSH above 2 and complaining of hypothyroid symptoms (depression, fatigue, brain fog, etc.) should be placed on thyroid hormone.

While doctors have been debating the numbers, millions of low thyroid patients have gone improperly diagnosed and untreated.

To complicate matters, the parameters for determining thyroid disorder have recently changed. The new guidelines narrow the range for acceptable thyroid function to 0.3–3.04. The AACE believes that the new range will result in proper diagnoses for millions of Americans who suffer from a mild thyroid disorder but have gone untreated until now. At a press conference in 2004, Hossein Gharib, MD, FACE, and president of AACE, said: "This means that there are more people with minor thyroid abnormalities than previously perceived." And how! The AACE estimates that the new guidelines actually double the number of people who have abnormal thyroid function, bringing the total to as many as 27 million.[5]

Even though there has been some progress, I still routinely receive test results that use the old numbers, and unfortunately many doctors continue to misdiagnose their patients based on these outdated lab parameters.

I've always advocated treating a patient and her symptoms instead of just her blood work. Many of my patients with pronounced low thyroid symptoms have normal blood tests. Blood tests for thyroid function are simply a poor diagnostic tool.

What is interesting is that some of my patients who presented to their medical doctor a year ago and had a TSH of 4 were told they were normal. Now if they go back to this same doctor (under the current guidelines), they'll be diagnosed as being hypothyroid. Clearly there is still some confusion about blood TSH levels.

EUTHYROID SYNDROME

Euthyroid is a medical term for patients who have normal thyroid blood tests but have all the symptoms associated with hypothyroidism: fatigue, low metabolism, headache, etc. Euthyroid patients may have a problem with T4 converting into active T3; their blood tests may not show this unless their doctor orders a special reverse T3 study. (because stress or chronic illness can cause T4 to change into reverse T3 instead of the active form of T3.) Individuals might then be put on synthetic thyroid hormones (like Synthroid, which contains T4 only), but since the T4 is not converting efficiently, they continue to have the symptoms of low thyroid.

Selenium is needed to convert T4 to T3, so a selenium deficiency can cause thyroid dysfunction. High blood levels of fatty acids (blood fats or triglycerides) can also inhibit conversion of T4 to T3.[6]

Patients often relate that they, and sometimes their doctors, suspected a thyroid problem only to have their blood work return normal. Most physicians, in this case, won't recommend thyroid replacement therapy. Many don't know about (or they choose to ignore) well documented studies that show that low body temperature is indicative of euthyroid hypothyroidism.

SELF-TEST FOR LOW THYROID

Dr. Broda Barnes was the first to show that a low basal body temperature was associated with low thyroid. His first study was published in 1942 and appeared in *JAMA*. This study tracked 1,000 college students and showed that monitoring body temperature for thyroid function was a valid if not superior approach to other thyroid tests.

The test for low thyroid function, according to Dr. Barnes's protocol, starts first thing in the morning. While still in bed, shake down and place the thermometer (preferably mercury; digital thermometers are not as accurate) under your arm and leave it there for 10 minutes. Record your temperature in a daily log. Women who are still having menstrual cycles should take their temperature after the third day of their period. Menopausal women can take their temperature on any day. A reading below the normal 98.2° strongly suggests hypothyroid. A reading above 98.2° may indicate hyperthyroidism (overactive thyroid).[7]

The body works best at the optimal temperature of 98.6°. Higher temperatures (fevers) speed up the metabolism and allow the body to fight off infection. A temperature of 90° or below qualifies as hypothermia, a medical emergency. But it doesn't have to go that low to affect health, because most of the biochemical reactions that occur in the body are driven by enzymes, and these enzymes are influenced by metabolic temperature.

Nutrition is involved in every aspect of T4 production, utilization, and conversion to triiodthyronine T3. The mineral zinc, along with iodine, vitamins A, B2, B3, B6, and C, as well as the amino acid tyrosine are all needed for the production of thyroxine (T4) hormone.[8]

Iodine and the amino acid derivative, h-tyrosine are direct precursors for thyroxine T4. A deficiency in either one of these nutrients can lead to thyroid dysfunction.

THE BARNES METHOD

Dr. Barnes recommends patients take a desiccated thyroid glandular medication known as Armour Thyroid, which was used before synthetic medications such as Synthroid were introduced. Armour Thyroid and other prescription thyroid glandulars (including Westhroid), contain both T4 and T3.[9]

Synthroid and many other synthetic thyroid medications contain T4 only. (Thyrolar contains T4 and T3). Since some individuals have a difficult time converting inactive T4 to active T3, these medications may not work at the cellular level. Individuals may take T4 medications for years and never notice much improvement. For many patients, of course, synthetic medications are adequate and sometimes preferable. For other patients, however, synthetic medications don't relieve all their symptoms, while desiccated thyroid does.

Most doctors believe T4 has no problem converting to T3 and therefore prescribe only synthetic T4 medication (such as Synthroid, Levoxyl, Levothroid, Eltroxin, Unithroid, and others). If the thyroid gland is malfunctioning and not producing enough—or any—T4, why assume that it still is capable of converting enough of its T4 to T3? Research continues to show that T4, administered *along with* T3, yields the best clinical outcome for many patients, especially those suffering from mood disorders.

LOW THYROID AND DEPRESSION

Depressed patients often benefit by taking T3 with or without their antidepressant medications.[10] Thyroid replacement therapy, especially the addition of T3, helps increases the effectiveness of tricyclic antidepressant medications.[11] Studies show that T3 therapy is more effective in reducing the symptoms associated with depression than SSRI antidepressants.[12]

Consider a report by three psychiatric researchers from the Department of Psychiatry, University of Toronto. They studied nine depressed thyroid-disease patients on T4-replacement therapy. Adding T3 to their therapy improve the patients' depression. The depression of seven of the nine patients (78%) decreased by at least 50%![13]

Dr. Ridha Arem, MD, author of *The Thyroid Solution,* agrees that "Increasing evidence indicates that T3, the most active form of thyroid hormone, is an effective antidepressant, when used in conjunction with a conventional antidepressant." A study by the *New England Journal of Medicine* showed that patients who received a combination of T4 and T3 were mentally sharper, less depressed, and feeling better overall than a control group who received T4 only.[14]

Unfortunately, even though T3 and combination T4-T3 therapy have been shown to help reduce depression, many doctors still use synthetic T4 medications exclusively.[15]

T3 has improved or eliminated depression, brain fog, feeling cold, constipation, chronic fatigue, headaches, insomnia, muscle and joint pain, and chronic sinus infections. For some people it has helped them finally lose weight.

Pharmaceutical company representatives typically report that synthetic medications for hypothyroidism are superior to desiccated thyroid.

They falsely accuse desiccated thyroid as being unstable or unpredictable. Since these sales representatives are the primary source of information about drugs for most doctors, this myth is passed from doctor to patient. But unlike desiccated thyroid, synthetic medications have often been recalled due to batch inconsistencies. Armour Thyroid conducts analytical tests on the thyroid powder (raw material) and on the actual tablets (finished product) to assure consistency in the T4 and T3 activity.

WILSON'S SYNDROME

Wilson's syndrome was first described by E. Denis Wilson, MD. He was refining some of the pioneering clinical research first performed by Dr. Barnes. Dr. Wilson showed that symptoms of low thyroid function could be present with normal thyroid blood tests. The group of symptoms that he studied he called Wilson's syndrome.

These symptoms can include severe fatigue, headache and migraine, PMS, easy weight gain, fluid retention, irritability, anxiety, panic attacks, depression, decreased memory and concentration, hair loss, decreased sex drive, unhealthy nails, constipation, irritable bowel syndrome, dry skin, dry hair, cold and/or heat intolerance, low self-esteem, irregular periods, chronic or repeated infections, and many other complaints.

Perhaps the greatest obstacle Dr. Wilson has had to overcome in his attempts to be recognized by mainstream medicine is the vast symptoms associated with Wilson's Syndrome. Yet all these symptoms can be seen in hypothyroid patients.

STRESS LEADS TO WILSON'S SYNDROME

The symptoms tend to come on or become worse after a major stressful event. Childbirth, divorce, death of a loved one, job or family stress, chronic illness, surgery, trauma, excessive dieting, and other stressful events can all lead to hypothyroidism.

Under significant physical, mental, or emotional stress the body slows down the metabolism by decreasing the amount of raw material (T4) that is converted to the active thyroid hormone (T3). This is done to conserve energy. However, when the stress is over, the metabolism is supposed to speed up and return to normal. This process can become derailed by a buildup of rT3 hormone. Reverse T3 can build to such high levels that it begins to start using up the enzyme that converts T4 to T3. The body may try to correct this by releasing more TSH and T4 only to have the levels of rT3 go even higher. A vicious cycle is created where T4 is never converted into active T3.

Certain nationalities are more likely to develop Wilson's syndrome: those whose ancestors survived famine, such as Irish, American Indian, Scotch, Welsh, and Russian. Interestingly, those patients who are part Irish and part American Indian are the most prone of all. Women are also more likely than men to develop Wilson's syndrome.

TESTING FOR WILSON'S SYNDROME

Like with Dr. Barnes's protocol, patients suspected of Wilson's syndrome monitor their body temperature. Those with Wilson's syndrome have temperatures that run below 98°, with 97.8° being typical. The temperature is taken three–four times daily over a five–seven day period. Patients are instructed to shake down and place a thermometer (preferably mercury) under their tongue for 10 minutes. An average day's temperature plotted over five–seven days will reveal if Wilson's syndrome is present.

TREATMENT OF WILSON'S SYNDROME

The way the cycle of Wilson's syndrome is stopped and the problem corrected is by reducing the rT3 levels so that T4 can convert to active T3.

A specially compounded form of timed-released T3 is used in gradual increments. T3 is available as a separate synthetic medication with the brand name Cytomel in the US and Canada, and Tertroxin in the UK. It's usually prescribed along with a synthetic T4 medication.

Body temperature is monitored, and when it returns to normal, the patients gradually wean themselves off the medicine. A big advantage of this over other hormone replacement therapies is that Wilson's syndrome patients are usually able to correct their low thyroid problem and eventually discontinue the medicine.

Wilson's protocol can be hard for patients to follow, but it often yields results when Armour and Westhroid therapies fail. I've used both protocols and gotten dramatic results for many of my patients. Some of my patients have been on synthetic thyroid medications for years with very little or no improvement. So I'm often amazed at the turnaround they experience when starting this program. Many of them enjoy a newfound energy and metabolism, and it's common for them to lose weight that couldn't be lost before, to sleep better, to rid themselves of chronic infections, and to think clearly for the first time in years.

GLANDULAR THYROID SUPPLEMENTS

I prefer that my patients take Armour Thyroid. However, if your doctor is reluctant to prescribe this due to your normal thyroid blood tests, over-the-counter thyroid glandular supplements are also available. These come from pig glands just like Armour Thyroid does. But they contain no T4, only T3. By removing the T4, manufacturers are able to legally sell the glandular extract without a prescription. These OTC medications can be used as a first line of treatment for low to moderate hypothyroid dysfunction.

Thyroid glandular supplements can be found online, in your local healthfood store, or by calling my office. I've been very pleased with Biotics Research's thyroid glandular supplements. I've been using them for almost two years, and my patients report that they feel better and notice improved energy, better moods, increased mental clarity, and needed weight loss on these supplements.

DOSING

I start my low-thyroid patients on one tablet twice a day of Biotics Research (which has 20 mg. of T3 glandular extract) glandular supplement. Then I have patients monitor their basal or oral temperatures (preferably with a mercury thermometer). After two weeks, if your temperature is not going up, or you're not feeling better, increase your dose to two tablets in the morning and one in the afternoon. Continue to monitor your temperatures.

If your temperature doesn't go up or you don't feel any better while using thyroid glandular supplementation, try adding Biotics Research's Cytozyme PT/HPT. This supplement helps increase the effectiveness of T3 glandular supplements. It can be ordered by calling my office or through your nutrition-oriented physician.

For information on ordering thyroid replacement supplements please see Appendix B.

RESOURCES

- www.wilsonssyndrome.com
- www.brodabarnes.org
- *Hypothyroidism: The Unsuspected Illness* by Broda Barnes, MD, and Lawrence Galton; 1976
- *Wilson's Thyroid Syndrome* by Denis Wilson, MD; 1991

1. *Life Extension Foundation's Disease Prevention and Treatment Protocols,* 3rd edition.
2. ibid.
3. ibid.
4. Kraus RP, Phoenix E, Edmonds E, Nicholson IR, Chandarana PC, Tokmakejian S. "Exaggerated TSH Responses to TRH in Depressed Patients With 'Normal' Baseline TSH." *J Clin Psychiatry* 1997;58:266-270.
5. As reported on the AACE website 2003.
6. Suzuki, Y. et al. "Plasma free fatty acids, inhibitor of extra thyroid conversion of T4 to T3 and thyroid hormone binding inhibitor in patients with various nonthyroid illnesses." *Endocrinol Jpn* 39(5). 445–53, 1992.
7. *Hypothyroidism: The Unsuspected Illness* by Broda Barnes, MD, and Lawrence Galton; 1976.
8. Arem, R., *The Thyroid Solution,* Ballantine Books, 1999, New York. also Shames, RL, Shames, KH, *Thyroid Power: 10 Steps to Total Health,* Harper Collins Publishers, New York, 2001. See: www.ThyroidPower.com and Brownstein, D., *Overcoming Thyroid Disorders,* Medical Alternatives Press, 2002. See: http://www.drbrownstein.com/
9. See 7 above.
10. Cooke RG, Joffe RT, Levitt AJ. "T3 augmentation of antidepressant treatment in T4-replaced thyroid patients." *J Clin Psychiatry* 1992 Jan;53(1):16-8.
11. Altshuler LL, Bauer M, Frye MA, et al. "Does thyroid supplementation accelerate tricyclic antidepressant response? A review and meta-analysis of the literature." *Am J Psychiatry* 2001 Oct;158(10):1617-22.
12. Agid O, Lerer B. "Algorithm-based treatment of major depression in an outpatient clinic: clinical correlates of response to a specific serotonin reuptake inhibitor and to triiodothyronine augmentation." *Int J Neuropsychopharmacol* 2003 Mar;6(1):41-49.
13. See 11 above.
14. From *A Clinician's View of Biotics Research Products,* a lecture by Harry O. Eidenier, Jr., Ph.D. July 2003.
15. Gaby, A. MD. " 'Sub-laboratory' Hypothyroidism and Empirical Use of Armour Thyroid." *Altern Med Rev* 2004; 9(2): 157–79.

9

Vitamins, Minerals, Herbals, and Mood

Vitamins and minerals help the brain make

needed neurotransmitters. Unfortunately,

most physicians do not prescribe natural

supplements to treat depression.

Some well-meaning yet woefully misinformed doctors may tell you that you don't need nutritional supplements. Yet numerous studies published in the very journals these physicians are reading demonstrate the need for vitamin and mineral supplementation. Deficiencies in magnesium, chromium, zinc, and other nutrients are common in our society. And in many cases, depressed people with blood levels indicating that they lack key nutrients respond quite well to supplements.[1]

Almost as criminal as not recommending vitamin and mineral supplements is the recommendation of them based on the government's recommended daily allowance (RDA). The RDA is some 50 years out of date. It was never intended to advance health, only to prevent diseases like scurvy and rickets. When was the last time you heard of anyone having these diseases? Taking the minimum amount of a nutrient might prevent you from getting scurvy, but it doesn't help those people who want to enjoy optimal health.

Making recommendations based on the RDA is like traveling in a horse and buggy when you could be riding in a Cadillac. Sure, the horse will probably get you where you want to go, but why not get around in comfort and style? Just about everyone could benefit from taking a good multivitamin, one based on the RDA but the ODA *(optimal* daily allowance). The ODA is based on clinical trials, experience, and other nutritionally-oriented physicians, including James Braly, MD.[2] (See page 35 for more about the RDA.)

The benefits of taking a good multivitamin/mineral formula on a daily basis have been reported in medical journals, popular newspapers, and magazines. Doing so reduces the incidence of heart disease, heart attack, stroke, glaucoma, macular degeneration, type-2 diabetes, senile dementia, and various cancers. The chart below compares the RDA to the ODA of a few select vitamins and minerals. (IU stands for international unit.)

	RDA	**ODA**
Vitamin A	1,000 mcg.	10,000 mg.
Vitamin D	200 IU	100 IU
Vitamin E	15 IU	400 IU
Vitamin K	80 mcg.	60–80 mcg.
Vitamin B1	1.5 mg.	50 mg–100mg.
Vitamin B2	1.7 mg.	50 mg.
Vitamin B3	19 mg.	50 mg.
Vitamin B5	7 mg.	200 mg.–400 mg.
Vitamin B6	2 mg.	50mg.–200 mg.
Folic Acid	200 mcg.	400–800 mcg.
Vitamin C	60 mg.	1,000–2, 0000 mg.
Calcium	800 mg.	500–1,200 mg.
Chloride	750 mg.	Not usually recommended
Chromium	50–200 mcg.	200–400 mcg.
Copper	1.5–3.0 mg.	1 mg.
Fluoride	1.5–4.0 mg.	Not usually recommended
Iodine	150 mcg.	Not usually recommended
Iron	10 mg.	Not unless needed
Magnesium	350 mg.	500–1,000 mg.
Manganese	2.5–5.0 mg.	10–20 mg.
Molybdenum	75–250 mcg.	Same (unless deficient)
Phosphorus	800 mg.	Not usually recommended
Potassium	2,000 mg.	100 mg.
Selenium	70 mcg.	200 mcg.
Sodium	500 mg.	Not usually recommended
Zinc	15 mg.	25 mg.

Vitamins and minerals play an important role in preventing and reversing the ill effects of anxiety and depression. For instance, neurotransmitters depend on adequate amounts of B vitamins in order to join with the amino acids tryptophan, glutamine and phenylalanine to make serotonin, GABA, dopamine, and norepinephrine.

THOSE BEAUTIFUL Bs

B vitamins are so important for producing and maintaining optimal neurotransmitters that a deficiency in any of the B vitamins can lead to host of symptoms associated with anxiety and depression disorders. Too-low levels have been linked to depression and bipolar disorder in a number of studies. Insufficient folic acid is one of the most common nutritional deficiencies, and one third of depressed adults are low in it. A deficiency of vitamin B12 can also lead to inadequate amounts of acetylcholine, an important neurotransmitter involved in learning and memory.

Folic acid is needed for the creation of the catecholamines, including dopamine, norepinephrine, and epinephrine.[3,4,5] It's also involved with energy production, synthesis of DNA, formation of red blood cells, and metabolism of all amino acids. A deficiency in folic acid (one the most common vitamin deficiencies), can produce macrocytic anemia, digestive disorders, heart palpitations, unhealthy weight loss, poor appetite, headaches, irritability, depression, insomnia, and mood swings. (A sore, red tongue may indicate a folic acid deficiency.) In addition, folic acid needs vitamins B12, B3 and C to be converted into its active form.

Folic acid can improve birth weight and neurological development in infants *and* prevent neural tube defects when taken by a pregnant mother. Women who are trying to get pregnant and expectant mothers should take a multi-vitamin with at least 400 mcg. of folic acid.

FOLIC ACID (VITAMIN B9)

But folate isn't only for pregnant women! Several studies have demonstrated the effectiveness of folic acid in reversing depression. One of these studies evaluated the use of folic acid supplementation in a group of patients suffering from depression or schizophrenia. Results showed that 92% of the folic acid group made a full recovery, compared with only 70% of the control group who took the standard prescription drug therapy. Those who received the folic acid spent only 23 days in the hospital, while those on prescription therapy alone averaged 33 hospital days.[6,7] One British study shows that depressed individuals with low folic acid were often poor responders to prescription antidepressant drug therapy. The addition of folic acid increased the recovery time of these depressed individuals.[8]

Another study showed that women who received folic acid plus Prozac had a greater reduction in depression symptoms that women who took Prozac alone. The women who took 400 mcg. of folic acid also reduced their blood levels of homocysteine.[9] Although this study didn't show any change in men who took folic acid along with Prozac compared to Prozac alone, studies show that men often need to double the amount of folic acid used in this study. The women in the study too 500 mcg. of folic acid. I recommended that men with elevated homocysteine levels take between 800–1,000 mcg. of folic acid.

Folic acid deficiency alone can cause severe depression, as can vitamin B12 deficiency. A deficiency of any of several B vitamins, in fact, can cause depression as we'll see below. I encourage my patients to take a high potency multivitamin/mineral formula with a minimum of 800 mcg. of folic acid each day.

Warning: large doses (exceeding 1200 mcg. a day) of folic acid can mask a vitamin B12 deficiency.

THIAMIN (VITAMIN B1)

A deficiency thiamin may lead to beriberi, which causes confusion, high blood pressure, problems with the heart, and other symptoms. A less severe deficiency may produce anxiety, depression, fatigue, constipation, and numbness or a "pins-and-needles" sensation in the legs.

Thiamin is needed to metabolize carbohydrates, fats, and proteins. It is important for proper cell function, especially nerve cells. It is also involved in the production of acetylcholine, a nerve chemical directly related to memory energy (most physical and mental). A deficiency of thiamin can lead to fatigue, mental confusion, emaciation, depression, irritability, upset stomach, nausea, and tingling in the extremities. Thiamin deficiency has been reported in almost 50% of the elderly. Could this be one of the reasons pre-senile dementia and Alzheimer's disease have increased so dramatically over the past few decades?

Diets high in simple sugars, including alcohol, increase the chances of thiamin deficiency. The tannins in tea inhibit thiamin absorption.

Thiamine has resolved side effects of antidepressant medication, such as dry mouth, insomnia, and stomach upset—inexpensively and with no added side effects. Foods containing thiamine include kale, spinach, turnip greens, green peas, lettuce, cabbage, and many other vegetables.

I encourage my patients to take a high potency multivitamin/mineral formula with a minimum of 100 mg. of thiamine each day.

RIBOFLAVIN (VITAMIN B2)

Riboflavin is necessary for the metabolism of carbohydrates, fats, and proteins. It's found in the following foods: asparagus, broccoli, spinach, almonds, wheat germ, millet, and whole-wheat bread. It's also involved in producing the neurotransmitters—including serotonin, dopamine, GABA, and norepinephrine—responsible for sleeping, mental and physical energy, happiness, and mental acuity. A deficiency of riboflavin can cause soreness and burning of the lips, mouth, and tongue; sensitivity to light; itching and burning eyes; and cracks in the corners of the mouth. Riboflavin can help curb the craving for sweets and is needed for the synthesis of vitamin B6. Riboflavin is needed to convert the amino acid tryptophan to niacin (B3). Riboflavin may turn the urine a bright fluorescent yellow, but this only means that you're absorbing and then discarding any unused riboflavin.

I encourage my patients to take a high potency multivitamin/mineral formula with a minimum of 50–100 mg. of riboflavin a day.

NIACIN (VITAMIN B3)

Vitamin B3 is also known as niacin or niacinamide. This essential vitamin helps convert tryptophan into serotonin. Niacin plays an important role in mental health, and orthomolecular physicians have used niacin to treat schizophrenia, anxiety, and depression. This is because niacin is a by-product of the metabolism of tryptophan, and some psychiatric disorders are caused by a genetic inability to breakdown or absorb tryptophan. This inability can lead to aggressive behavior, restlessness, hyperactivity, and insomnia.

A deficiency of niacin causes weakness, dry skin, lethargy, headaches, irritability, loss of memory, depression, delirium, insomnia, and disorientation.

For the treatment of anxiety, depression, and insomnia, it is best to use a special version of vitamin B3 known as niacinamide, which won't cause flushing. Even mainstream medicine has begun to acknowledge its benefits. Hoffman LaRoche, the company that makes Valium, has reported that their research shows niacinamide acts like a benzodiazepine tranquilizer.[10] Fortunately niacinamide doesn't have the side effects associated with benzodiazepine drugs.

Individuals with a sluggish liver who take high doses of niacinamide may experience nausea. If this is troubling, discontinue niacinamide and begin taking the herb milk thistle, which helps optimize liver function. After a couple of weeks of taking milk thistle, add a low dose of niacinamide, and slowly increase the dose over a period of weeks. If the nausea returns, stop taking niacinamide.

Niacin or niacinamide acts as a wonderful sedative to calm nerves and help with sleep.

Warning: High doses of niacin may cause skin flushing. And timed-release niacin, often used to reduce high blood pressure, may cause elevated liver enzymes. Individuals with high blood pressure should take a special form of niacin known as inositol hexaniacinate or "no-flush" niacin. To reduce blood pressure, start with 400–500 mg. of no-flush niacin, and increase by 400–500 mg. every three days until blood pressure comes down or you reach a maximum dose of 4,000 mg. For more information about natural ways to reduce high blood pressure, see Appendix B to order my book *Heart Disease: What Your Doctor Won't Tell You.*

Foods that contain high levels of niacin include brewer's yeast, brown rice, whole wheat, seeds, nuts, peanuts, and other legumes. I encourage my patients to take a high potency multivitamin/mineral formula with a minimum 50–100 mg. of niacin a day. Some individuals may need to add an additional 500–1,000 mg. of niacinamide to their daily therapy.

PANTOTHENIC ACID (VITAMIN B5)

Pantothenic acid is needed to produce adrenal hormones, which play an important role in how well we deal with stress. In fact, pantothenic acid is sometimes referred to as the "anti-stress" vitamin. It can help reduce anxiety and may play a significant role in avoiding depression. It helps convert choline into acetylcholine, which is responsible for memory. A deficiency can lead to fatigue, depression, irritability, digestive problems, upper respiratory infections, dermatitis, muscle cramps, and loss of sensation in the extremities.

Pantothenic acid is needed by all cells in the body, especially those of the gastrointestinal tract. It converts carbohydrates, fats, and proteins into energy and, along with vitamin C, helps to reduce uric acid levels. (Increased uric acid levels are associated with gouty arthritis.) Pantothenic acid helps boost endurance by manufacturing ATP, an essential chemical for cellular energy.

Warning: Large doses may cause diarrhea.

Pantothenic acid is found in most leafy green vegetables and whole grain foods. I encourage my patients to take a high potency multivitamin/mineral formula with a minimum 200–500 mg. of B5 a day.

PYRIDOXINE (VITAMIN B6)

Pyridoxine, better known as B6, is needed to convert the amino acids into their respective brain chemical. It may be the most important B vitamin, since it is involved in more bodily functions than any other vitamin. B6 is crucial for making neurotransmitters and inhibits the formation of homocysteine (the toxic chemical we already discussed on page 44). It is involved in the synthesis of DNA and RNA, which make up the genetic blueprint of cells. It helps metabolize essential fatty acids and, as a major antioxidant, helps prevent the destruction caused by free radicals. It helps produce hydrochloric acid, which is crucial for proper digestion, and the formation of hemoglobin is dependent on it.

A B6 deficiency can cause anemia, even if normal iron levels are present. A deficiency can also cause depression, insomnia, fatigue, tingling and numbness in the extremities, increased susceptibility to infections, nausea, kidney stones, and anemia. It can be suppressed by certain medications, including oral contraceptives and estrogen. Symptoms associated with a B6 deficiency include premenstrual syndrome, depression, irritability, tension, headaches, fluid retention, and acne; these can be reduced by supplementation. B6 can also serve as a natural diuretic or alleviate carpal tunnel syndrome. It is also needed for proper magnesium levels in red blood cells.

Some asthmatics have a malfunction in the way they assimilate pyridoxine and process tryptophan. Supplementing with 250–500 mg. of pyridoxine daily can help alleviate asthma symptoms.

B6 is found in brewer's yeast, sunflower seeds, soybeans, walnuts, lentils, lima beans, hazelnuts, brown rice, avocados, and many other common foods. Therefore, deficiencies are not common. However, depending on a person's unique biochemical needs, low B6 levels can lead to depression, poor nerve function, carpel tunnel syndrome, and other problems. Alcoholics and women who are pregnant, lactating, or taking oral contraceptives are prone to developing a B6 deficiency.

Also prone to B6 deficiency are those suffering from **pyroluria,** a genetic disorder that creates a group of chemicals known as kryptopyrroles. These chemicals may be found in as many as 40% of those suffering from a mood disorder.[11] Normally a harmless by-product of hemoglobin metabolism, little if any kryptopyrroles a circulating in the blood of healthy individuals. These chemicals bind to aldehyde chemicals and block the absorption and utilization of pyridoxine. This process causes zinc to become deficient as well, and it's a recipe for disaster in those with an already bankrupt stress-coping savings account.

Individuals suffering from pyroluria may have some of these characteristics: fair skin that sunburns easily, lack of dreaming at night, history of cluster headaches, PMS, anemia, cold hands or feet, tingling sensations in the hands or feet, motion sickness, poor immune function (lots of colds, flu's or infections each year), white spots on the fingernails, stretch marks on the skin, sensitivity to sunlight, and dislike of protein-rich foods. All of these suggest a B6 or zinc deficiency.

There are tests for detecting pyroluria, which I recommend for patients who aren't making the expected progress fast enough. See Appendix B for more information on these tests. Those with pyroluria will often be also suffering from adrenal fatigue.

I encourage my patients to take a high potency multivitamin/mineral formula with a minimum of 100 mg. of B6 daily. Some individuals have trouble converting B6 into the more active pyridoxil-5-phosphate (P5P), so I recommend taking a combination of B6 and P5P.

COBALAMIN (VITAMIN B12)

A vitamin B12 deficiency can lead to a host of unwanted symptoms including pernicious anemia, anxiety, depression, fatigue, and poor mental function. B12 is responsible in the replication of the genetic material in all the cells and therefore is essential for the development and maintenance of all cells. It also helps form the myelin sheath that insulates nerve processes. This sheath allows rapid communication from one cell to another. So a deficiency can cause a reduction in mental acuity, evidenced by poor memory.

B12 inhibits monoamine oxidase (MAO), an enzyme that metabolizes some of the neurotransmitters that help to elevate mood. Because of this, it acts like an MAO inhibitor drug (MAOI) prescribed for depression. However, unlike MAOIs, B12 doesn't have negative side effects.

Although B12 deficiency is not as common as folic acid deficiency, it is more common than many people—including doctors—suspect. Even low normal levels can contribute to depression, particularly in the elderly.

A small but significant number of senior citizens have difficulty absorbing B12 from their food. This may be from taking stomach-acid blocking medications—such as Prevacid, Tagamet, Zantac, and Nexium—or from a deficiency of intrinsic factor, a substance needed for proper B12 absorption. So I believe everyone over the age of 60 should be taking extra B12. Anti-gout medications, anti-coagulant drugs, and potassium supplements may interfere with B12 absorption.

Alzheimer's and senile dementia, associated with memory loss, confusion, and nerve damage, can both occur due to a deficiency of B12. Calcium is necessary for normal absorption of B12.

B12 is found in most animal products, including beef liver, chicken liver, clams, oysters, and sardines, with smaller amounts in eggs, many fish, and cheeses. Vegetarians run the risk of becoming B12 deficient and should definitely supplement their diet with B12.

It is best to take a sublingual (melts under the tongue) form of B12, especially if you're suffering from pernicious anemia, anxiety, or depression. My patients, however, often take a high potency multivitamin/mineral formula with a minimum 100 mcg. of B12 daily. Those with anxiety and or depression may need to supplement with extra sublingual B12.

CHOLINE

Choline, with the help of vitamin B5, is converted by the body into the neurotransmitter acetylcholine, which plays an important role in learning and memory. Our bodies can make choline from vitamin B12, folic acid, and an amino acid, methionine. Choline is essential for brain development and proper liver function. A deficiency in choline may cause poor memory and mental fatigue.

Foods high in choline include eggs, brewer's yeast, soybeans, green peas, and peanuts. I encourage my patients to take a high potency multivitamin/mineral formula with a minimum 300 mcg. of choline a day.

BIOTIN (VITAMIN H, VITAMIN Bw)

Biotin is a water soluble vitamin critical to the body's fat metabolism, and it aids in the utilization of protein, folic acid, cobalamin, and pantothenic acid . Symptoms of a deficiency include depression, dry skin, brittle nails, conjunctivitis, hair loss and hair color loss, elevated cholesterol, anemia, loss of appetite, muscle pain, numbness in the hands and feet, nausea, lethargy, and enlargement of the liver. Sufficient quantities are needed for healthy hair and nails. Biotin may help prevent hair loss in some men. It is also important in promoting healthy bone marrow, nervous tissue, and sweat glands.

The artificial sweetener saccharin inhibits the absorption of biotin. Raw egg whites, antibiotics, and sulfa drugs all prevent proper utilization of biotin. Due to poor absorption, infants are susceptible to a biotin deficiency; symptoms include a dry, scaly scalp and face (known as seborrheic dermatitis). Biotin deficiencies are rare and usually seen in hospitalized patients on intravenous feeding tubes or in patients taking large dosages of antibiotics.

I encourage my patients to take a high potency multivitamin/mineral formula with a minimum of 300 mcg. of biotin daily.

CALCIUM

Calcium is the most abundant mineral in the body. It comprises some two–three pounds of total body weight, and is essential for the formation of bones and teeth. Calcium contributes to the release of neurotransmitters, and it can have a calming affect on the nervous system. It regulates heart rhythm, cellular metabolism, muscle coordination, blood clotting, and nerve transmission. Adequate intake of calcium can help lower high blood pressure and the incidence of heart disease. A deficiency of calcium can result in hypertension, insomnia, osteoporosis, muscle spasm, and periodontal disease.

Calcium also depends on other nutrients for maximum benefit. The body prefers a calcium-to-magnesium ratio of 1.5- or 2-to-1 and a calcium-to-phosphorous ratio of 2- or 3-to-1. Vitamin D is also required for the absorption of calcium.

Calcium absorption is decreased by junk food (high protein, fat, and phosphorous) diets. Chelated calcium (bound to a protein for easier absorption) and magnesium can help reduce aluminum and lead poisoning.

Warning: Excessive calcium intake (several grams a day) can cause calcium deposits in the soft tissue, including the blood vessels (where they cause arteriosclerosis) and kidneys (where they cause stones). Oyster shell or bone meal calcium supplements often contain high levels of toxic lead. Supplement with calcium citrate or calcium ascorbate instead.

I encourage my patients to take a high potency multivitamin/mineral formula with a minimum 500–1200 mg. of calcium daily.

CHROMIUM

Chromium is essential in the synthesis of cholesterol, fats, and protein. It also helps stabilize blood sugar and insulin levels; abnormal levels have been shown to contribute to brain fog, mental fatigue, anxiety, and depression. Proper interaction between blood sugar and insulin ensures proper protein production, reducing the chance for fat storage.

A deficiency in chromium can cause type-2 diabetes, hypoglycemia, and coronary artery disease. Estimates are that 90% of the U S population is deficient in chromium! Diets high in simple sugars increase the loss of chromium, and a deficiency can cause a craving for sugar.

I encourage my patients to take a high potency multivitamin/mineral formula with a minimum of 200–400 mcg. of chromium each day.

INOSITOL

An unofficial member of the B vitamin family, inositol is present in all tissues, with the highest levels in the brain and heart. It functions closely with choline and is also a component of cell membranes. The proper action of several neurotransmitters, including serotonin and acetylcholine, requires inositol. It's important in the metabolism of fats and cholesterol and in the proper function of the kidneys and liver. It is also vital for hair growth and prevents hardening of the arteries. Inositol is needed for the synthesis of lecithin, which helps remove fats from the liver. Along with the amino acid GABA, inositol may help reduce anxiety. Caffeine may decrease inositol stores.

Various studies have found that inositol benefits people with depression. One study showed that individuals with moderate to severe depression who consumed 12 g. of inositol each day significantly reduced their anxiety and depression.[12,13,14] I routinely find that my patients benefit from a more modest 1,000–2,000 mg. (1–2 g.) of powdered inositol.

I encourage my patients to take a high potency multivitamin/mineral formula with a minimum of 25 mg. of inositol daily. Larger doses may be needed for those suffering from anxiety disorder.

VITAMIN D

Vitamin D is considered both a vitamin and a hormone, since our bodies, when exposed to sunlight, can produce it. During winter months, when the days are shorter and many folks spend less time outdoors, vitamin D can become deficient, leading some individuals to develop seasonal affective disorder (SAD). SAD can be treated with vitamin D supplementation.[15]

Bright light therapy is another way to reverse the symptoms of SAD.

I encourage my patients to take a high potency multivitamin/mineral formula with a minimum 400–800 IU of vitamin D daily.

VITAMIN C (ASCORBIC ACID)

Vitamin C acts as an antioxidant and helps to maintain the immune system, manufacture collagen, guard against cancer and heart disease, reduce the risk of cataracts, and otherwise encourage health. A deficiency can lead to depression and mental confusion, among other problems. In fact, depression is the first clinical symptom detected when humans are deliberately deprived of vitamin C. Vitamin C is important in the conversion of tryptophan to serotonin. And, as you know so well by now, low serotonin levels are linked to insomnia and depression.

A deficiency of vitamin C causes an increase in urinary excretion of vitamin B6, which is also associated with making neurotransmitters. Vitamin C helps prevent toxicity from heavy metals including cadmium, mercury, and lead. Such toxicity has been linked to an increased risk of heart disease and mood disorders. Aspirin, alcohol, antidepressants, anti-coagulants, oral contraceptives, analgesics, and steroids can all interfere with vitamin C absorption.

One study found that women who attempted suicide had lower levels of vitamin C than those who had not. And when researchers compared the amount of vitamin C in the blood of 885 psychiatric patients and 110 healthy controls, the psychiatric patients were found to have significantly lower levels.[16]

Vitamin C produces and maintains collagen, a protein that forms the foundation for connective tissue, the most abundant tissue in the body. Vitamin C is important in fighting bacterial infections, healing wounds, preventing hemorrhaging, reducing allergy symptoms, and helping to prevent heart disease. A potent antioxidant, it helps prevent free radical damage. A natural antihistamine, it can reduce blood pressure in mild hypertension. It prevents the progression of cataracts, helps regulate blood sugar levels, works to regulate cholesterol so that it is excreted out of the body, and may help improve fertility. It increases the immune system function, and is involved in the formation of important stress hormones produced by the adrenal glands.

A deficiency in vitamin C can cause bleeding gums; loose teeth; dry, scaly skin; tender joints; muscle cramps; poor wound healing; lethargy; loss of appetite; depression; and swollen arms and legs.

Foods high in vitamin C include red chili peppers, guava, parsley, green and sweet red peppers, broccoli, strawberries, oranges, mangoes, and cantaloupe. Most vitamin C is lost in the urine, but Ester C is absorbed four times faster than regular ascorbic acid. So much less is lost in urination.

I encourage my patients to take a high potency multivitamin/mineral formula with a minimum 1,000–2,000 mg. of vitamin C daily.

Warning: Pregnant women should not exceed 5,000 mg. of vitamin C in a day. Large doses may also cause loose stools or diarrhea.

COPPER

Copper maintains the myelin sheath, which wraps around nerves and facilitates nerve communication. It plays a vital role in regulating the neurotransmitters and an integral part in maintaining the cardiovascular and skeletal systems. It is part of the antioxidant enzyme supraoxide dismutase and may help protect cells from free radical damage. Copper helps with the absorption of iron, and a deficiency in copper can lead to anemia, gray hair, heart disease, poor concentration, numbness and tingling in the extremities, decreased immunity, and scoliosis.

The heavy metal cadmium interferes with copper absorption, and a niacin deficiency can cause an elevation of copper.

Warning: A daily intake of 20 mg. or more of copper can cause nausea and vomiting. Elevated levels of copper can cause paranoia, aggressiveness, hyperactivity, and premature aging. Wilson's disease is a genetic disorder characterized by excessive accumulation of copper in the tissues, liver disease, mental retardation, tremors, and loss of coordination.

I encourage my patients to take a high potency multivitamin/mineral formula with a minimum 1–2 mg. of copper daily.

POTASSIUM

Potassium is a mineral that helps to keep the heart beating regularly. Mental confusion, fatigue, and weakness—all symptoms of depression—have been associated with low levels of the mineral, and suicide victims usually show a deficiency of it. Maintaining adequate potassium levels helps to reverse the fatigue and muscle weakness that may be associated with depression, mental fatigue, or lethargy.

Foods high in potassium include bananas, nonfat milk, oranges, and fresh peas.

Eating four–five servings of fresh vegetables and fruit a day is usually enough to ensure an adequate amount of potassium. Still, I encourage my patients to take a high potency multivitamin/mineral formula with a minimum of 99 mg. of potassium daily.

MAGNESIUM

Magnesium plays a significant role in regulating the neurotransmitters. A deficiency in magnesium can cause depression, muscle cramps, high blood pressure, heart disease and arrhythmia, constipation, insomnia, loss of hair, confusion, personality disorders, swollen gums, and loss of appetite.

Magnesium is one of the most important minerals in the body. It is responsible for proper enzyme activity and the transmission of muscle and nerve impulses. It also aids in maintaining a proper pH balance and helps metabolize carbohydrates, proteins, and fats into energy. Magnesium helps synthesize the genetic material in cells and remove toxic substances (such as aluminum and ammonia) from the body.

A deficiency of magnesium may increase heart disease, as it works with calcium to ensure proper heart function. (Magnesium relaxes smooth muscles, including the heart, and calcium constricts or activates smooth muscle.)

Magnesium is a natural sedative and can be used to treat muscle spasm, anxiety, depression, insomnia, and constipation. It also helps with intermittent claudicating, a condition caused by a restriction of bloodflow to the legs. (For treatment, I recommend Bilberry and 600 mg. of magnesium). Magnesium is also effective in relieving some of the symptoms associated with premenstrual syndrome (PMS). Women who suffer from PMS are usually deficient in magnesium.

New studies are also finally validating what many nutrition-oriented physicians have known for years: a magnesium deficiency can trigger migraine headaches.

Magnesium helps relax constricted bronchial tubes associated with asthma. In fact, a combination of vitamin B6 and magnesium, along with avoidance of wheat and dairy products, has cured many of my young asthmatic patients.

High intake of calcium may reduce magnesium absorption, and simple sugars and stress deplete the body of magnesium. That's another reason to avoid simple sugars and stress; magnesium is a potent antidepressant!

I encourage my patients to take a high potency multivitamin/mineral formula with a minimum of 500 mg. of magnesium daily.

Warning: Symptoms of magnesium toxicity include nausea, lethargy, and difficulty in breathing. Magnesium supplemented above 600 mg. can cause loose stools and diarrhea in some individuals, but this is quickly remedied by decreasing the dosage.

MANGANESE

Manganese is needed in order to synthesize thiamin, and it works in coordination with the other B vitamins to reduce the effects of stress. A deficiency of manganese can cause fatigue, impaired fertility, retarded growth, birth defects, seizures, and bone malformations. It aids in the development of mother's milk and is important for normal bone and tissue growth. It is also involved in the production of cellular energy, metabolizes fats and proteins, and is essential in maintaining a healthy nervous system.

I encourage my patients to take a high potency multivitamin/mineral formula with a minimum of 10–20 mg. of manganese each day.

Warning: Elevated manganese may cause violent behavior, muscle spasm, and tremors.

SELENIUM

Selenium is an important antioxidant that protects the body from free-radical damage. It helps make thyroid hormones and essential fatty acids, and a deficiency in either of these increases the risk of developing anxiety and/or depression. Selenium is a component of glutathione peroxidase, an enzyme essential for detoxification of cellular debris. And it, along with other antioxidants (especially vitamin E), combats free radicals that can cause heart disease.

Warning: Doses above 600 mg. can cause side effects that include tooth decay and periodontal disease.

I encourage my patients to take a high potency multivitamin/mineral formula with a minimum of 200–400 mcg. of selenium daily.

ZINC

Zinc is important in over 90 enzymatic pathways. A zinc deficiency can cause depression, since it's necessary for the production of dopamine (one of the "happy hormones"). Zinc facilitates alcohol detoxification within the liver, and it plays a role in producing and digesting proteins. Zinc is also important in maintaining normal blood levels of vitamin A, boosting the immune system, healing wounds, converting calories to energy, reducing low birth rates and infant mortality, controlling blood cholesterol levels, and in producing the prostaglandin hormones that regulate heart rate, blood pressure, inflammation, mood disorders, and other processes.

A deficiency of zinc can lead to poor sense of taste, anorexia nervosa, anemia, depression, fatigue, increased pain, slow growth, birth defects, impaired nerve function, sterility, glucose intolerance, mental disorders, dermatitis, hair loss, and atherosclerosis.

Excess copper can cause a zinc deficiency, and vice versa. Women who are pregnant can accumulate excess copper and become zinc-deficient. And this can lead to post-partum depression. Extra zinc (50 mg. daily) should be consumed by pregnant females to help avoid post-partum depression.*

Zinc lozenges have been shown to reduce the symptoms and duration of colds by 50%. It is estimated that 68% of the population is deficient in zinc. White-speckled fingernails are indicative of a zinc deficiency.

I encourage my patients to take a high potency multivitamin/mineral formula with a minimum of 25 mg. of zinc daily.

DMAE

DMAE (dimethylaminoethanol) is a naturally occurring nutrient, found in sardines and other foods, that may help relieve depression and/or fatigue. A brain stimulant, DMAE passes through the blood-brain barrier into the brain, where it helps increase the levels of acetylcholine (a neurotransmitter that plays an important role in both mood and energy levels).

DMAE has been shown to elevate mood, improve memory and learning, and increase intelligence. It is even more effective when taken with vitamin B5 (pantothenate). DMAE has also been used with great success in the treatment of attention deficit disorder (ADD) in children and adults.

Depression often manifests itself as fatigue, so by directly increasing energy levels and through its ability to alleviate depression, DMAE attacks fatigue on two levels. See the next page for a summary of this nutrient's benefits.

---

*I don't recommend prescription prenatal vitamins for my pregnant patients, because they are insufficient in many nutrients. I instead recommend a high-potency multivitamin/mineral supplement, but with a maximum of 8,000 IU of vitamin A daily. More than that could run the risk of damaging the developing baby.

- increases physical energy
- decreases daytime fatigue and allows for more natural sleep at night
- is a safe antidepressant that elevates the mood
- increases the ability to learn (can even help raise IQ)
- helps reduce "brain debris" called lipofuscin, thereby improving brain function
- increases longevity as measured in laboratory animals

ST. JOHN'S WORT

In Germany, the herb St.John's Wort is covered by health insurance as a prescription drug, and some 20 million people take it for depression. Seventy percent of German physicians prefer to treat depression and anxiety with St. John's Wort. A review of 23 randomized double-blind placebo-controlled studies, involving 1757 people with mild or moderately severe depressive disorders, showed that St. John's Wort was nearly three times superior to a placebo in relieving depressive symptoms and was as effective as standard antidepressant drugs.[17]

One study revealed St. John's Wort (500 mg. a day) to be more effective then 20. mg a day of fluoxetine (Prozac) in reducing depression, and the herb produced significantly fewer incidences of side effects (8% of St. John's Wort patients versus 23% of Prozac patients).[18] Another study showed that St. John's Wort was as effective as 75 mg. twice a day of imipramine, again with far fewer side effects.[19]

The ideal dose of St. John's Wort is 300 mg. of standardized .3 hypericin. I usually don't start my patients on St. John's Wort initially. Instead I begin them on an ODA multivitamin/mineral formula with fish oil, free-form amino acids, and the appropriate amino-acid replacement therapy based on their Brain Function Questionnaire. If a patient isn't responding as quickly as I'd like, I add St. John's Wort.

I *don't* recommend that taking prescription antidepressant drugs take St. John's Wort.

MEDICATIONS CAN CAUSE DEFICIENCIES!

- **Aspirin** depletes folic acid, iron, potassium, sodium and vitamin C.
- **Beta-blockers** deplete coenzyme Q10 (co-Q10), an important nutrient for liver function and for cardiovascular and overall health. This can lead to heart disease, fatigue and muscle pain.
- **Amitriptyline (Elavil, Enovil)** depletes co-Q10 and vitamin B2.

This can cause headaches, anxiety, depression, heart disease, fatigue, and muscle pain.

- **Carbamazepine (Tegratol)** depletes biotin, folic acid, and vitamin D. This can cause pain, fatigue, and depression.
- **Celecoxib (Celebrex)** depletes folic acid.
- **Corticosteroids** (cortisone, dexamethasone, hydrocortisone, prednisone) depletes calcium, folic acid, magnesium, potassium, selenium, vitamin C, vitamin D, and zinc. This can cause depression, fatigue, pain, heart disease, and other illnesses.
- **Digoxin (Lanoxin)** depletes calcium, magnesium, phosphorus, and vitamin B1.
- **Estrogens** (Estrace, Estratab, Estrostep, Menest, Premarin) deplete magnesium, omega-3 fatty acids, vitamin B6, zinc, and omega-3 fatty acids. This can cause pain, depression, poor immune function, and other illnesses.
- **Famotidine (Pepcid and Pepcid AC)** depletes calcium, folic acid, iron, vitamin B12, vitamin D, and zinc. May lead poor immune function, fatigue, depression, and pain.
- **Hydrochlorothiazide** (Esidrix, Ezide, Dyazide, DydroDIURIL, Hydro-Par, Maxide, Microzide, Oretic) depletes co-Q10, magnesium, potassium, vitamin B6 and zinc.This could cause pain, fatigue, depression, restless leg syndrome, irritable bowel syndrome, spastic colon, and other illnesses.
- **NSAIDs** (fenoprofen, ibuprofen, neproxen, Aleve, Anaprox, Advil, Excedrin, Motrin, Naprosyn, Nuprin, Orudis, and Pamprin) deplete folic acid. This can cause anxiety and depression.
- **Omeprazole (Prilosec)** depletes vitamin B12. This can lead to fatigue, anemia, and depression.
- **Oral contraceptives** deplete vitamin C, vitamin B2, folic acid, magnesium, vitamin B6, vitamin B12 and zinc. This could lead to poor immune function, anxiety, depression, and fatigue.
- **Prevastatin (Pravachol)** depletes co-Q10. This could lead to heart disease, fatigue, and muscle pain.
- **Ranitidine hydrochloride (Zantac)** depletes calcium, folic acid, iron, vitamin B12, vitamin D, and zinc. This could cause poor immune function, fatigue, depression, anxiety, restless leg syndrome, anemia, and more.
- **Triamterine (Dyrenium)** depletes calcium, folic acid, and zinc. This could cause fatigue, depression, anxiety, and poor immunity.
- **Valproic acid (Depacote)** depletes carnitine and folic acid. This could contribute to diabetes, depression, and fatigue.
- **Statins** block production of co-Q10. This action can lead to muscle aches and pains.

1.Carney, M.W. "Neuropsychiatric disorders associated with nutritional deficiencies. Incidence and therapeutic implications." *CNS Drugs* 1995; 3(4): 279-90.

2.Keats Publishing, 1992.

3.Bukreev, "V.I. Effect of pyridoxine on the psychopathology and pathochemistry of involutional depressions." *Zh. Nevropatol. Psikhiatr. Im. S. S. Korsakova* 1978; 78(3): 402-8 (in Russian).

4.See 1 above.

5.Alpert, J.E., Fava, M. "Nutrition and depression: the role of folate." *Nutr. Rev.* 1997 May; 55(5): 145-9.

6.Kelly, G.S. "Folates: supplemental forms and therapeutic applications." *Altern. Med. Rev.* 1998 Jun; 3(3): 208-20.

7.See 1 above

8.Coppen, A., Bailey, J. "Enhancement of the antidepressant action of fluoxetine by folic acid: a randomized, placebo-controlled trial." *J. Affect. Disorders* 2000; 60: 121-30.

9.See 8 above

10.Joan Matthews Larsen, *Depression Free Naturally* Balletine Publishing, p. 156. New York, NY 1999.

11.See 10 above

12.Levine, J. "Controlled trials of inositol in psychiatry." *Eur. Neuropsychopharmacol.* 1997; 7(2): 147-55.

13.Levine, J., Barak, Y., Gonzalves, M., Szor, H., Elizur, A., Kofman, O., Belmaker, R.H. "Double-blind, controlled trial of inositol treatment of depression." *Am. J. Psychiatry* 1995a May; 152(5): 792-4.

14.Levine, J., Barak, Y., Kofman, O., Belmaker, R.H. "Follow-up and relapse analysis of an inositol study of depression." *Isr. J. Psychiatry Relat. Sci.* 1995b; 32(1): 14-21.

15.Lansdowne, A.T., Provost, S.C. "Vitamin D3 enhances mood in healthy subjects during winter." *Psychopharmacology* 1998 Feb; 135(4): 319-23.

16.Schorah, C.J., Morgan, D.B., Hullin, R.P. "Plasma vitamin C concentrations in patients in a psychiatric hospital." *Hum. Nutr. Clin. Nutr.* 1983 Dec; 37(6): 447-52.

17.Linde, K., Ramirez, G., Mulrow, C.D., Pauls, A., Weidenhammer, W., Melchart, D. "St. John's wort for depression-an overview and meta-analysis of randomised clinical trials." *Br. Med. J.* 1996 Aug 3; 313(7052): 253-8.

18.Schader, 2000

19.Woelk, H. "Comparison of St. John's wort and imipramine for treating depression: randomized controlled trial." *Br. Med. J.* 2000; 321: 536-9.

10

Lipids, EFAs, and Mood

The brain, nerves, reproductive organs, liver, and the

heart all have special lipids particularly designed for

each organ's optimal function. You need fat!

Lipids are substances that can't be dissolved in water. These include fats, oils, phospholipids (lecithin), and other substances made by the body. Fat, found in all natural foods, is an essential nutrient that plays a vital role in our overall health. We can't live without it. It provides energy, produces certain hormones, insulates us from cold, and makes up the cellular membranes. Fat is the primary source of fuel for the muscles (the heart included) and provides over twice the amount of energy of carbohydrates. A great deal of energy is needed just to keep the body warm, and fat provides 70% of this energy. The brain is 70% fat. It insulates the brain cells and allows the neurotransmitters to communicate with one another.

Cholesterol is a fat that helps keep cell membranes permeable. This permeability allows the good nutrients to get into the cell and the waste products to get out. Cholesterol is essential for proper brain function and normal neurotransmitter levels. A deficiency in cholesterol can result in mood disorders including depression, anxiety, irritability, and brain fog. Cholesterol is also involved in the production of such essential hormones as DHEA, testosterone, estradiol, progesterone, and cortisol.

Cholesterol is used by the body to repair and patch damaged cellular membranes. This is why scar tissue contains high levels of cholesterol and one of the reasons cholesterol is seen in arterial plaques. When an arterial cell is damaged from free radicals, infection, or other inflammatory processes, cholesterol is dispatched to patch the diseased tissue.

Because it is essential to our very survival, the body manufactures cholesterol on a daily basis. Only 15% of our cholesterol comes from food.

LOW CHOLESTEROL AND DEPRESSION

Several studies show that among older adults, those with low cholesterol are three times more likely to suffer from depression than those with normal cholesterol. And the lower the cholesterol, the more severe the depression.[1]

Low cholesterol levels are also linked to an increased risk of suicide. One study reported in the *British Medical Journal* showed that of the 300 people suicide victims studied, *all* showed low cholesterol levels.[2]

Men whose cholesterol levels are lowered through the use of prescription medication double their chances of committing suicide.[3]

ESSENTIAL FATTY ACIDS AND DEPRESSION

Fat is made up of fatty acids. The three major types of fatty acids are:

1. **Saturated fatty acids (SFAs)** are found in butter, coconut oil, eggs, meat, and cheese. Saturated fats consist of long, straight chains of molecules packed tightly together. Saturated fats are solid at room temperature.

2. **Monounsaturated fatty acids (MUFAs)** are found in almond oil, avocados, canola oil, oats, peanut oil, and olive oil. Monounsaturated oils are usually liquid at room temperature, but may become cloudy or hardened when placed in the refrigerator. MUFAs have one kink or bend in their structure and this makes them more flexible than SFAs.

3. **Polyunsaturated fatty acids (PUFAs)** are found in corn oil, primrose oil, flaxseed oil, borage oil, certain fish, sesame oil, sunflower, safflower, and wheat germ oil. Vegetable oils are usually high in PUFAs. Polyunsaturated fats (PUFAs) are liquid at room temperature. PUFAs have many kinks or bends in the chains of fatty acids

that make them up. These kinks or bends make PUFAs soft and flexible. PUFAs also make up our essential fatty acids (EFAs). Essential for our existence, EFAs cannot be manufactured by the body but must be obtained from the foods we eat. PUFAs are divided into two families of essential fatty acids (EFA).

- **Omega 6 linoleic acid.** Pure vegetable oils, including sunflower, safflower, and corn oil contain the essential fatty acid (EFA) Omega 6. Some individuals are genetically unable to convert Linoleic acid into its derivative, gamma linolenic acid (GLA). This can be overcome by taking primrose or borage oil; both are high in GLA.

- **Omega 3 linolenic acid.** Omega 3 oils including alpha linolenic acid (ALA) are found in flax seed, soybean, walnut, and chestnut oils, as well as some dark green leafy vegetables. Eicosapentaenoic acid (EPA) and DHA (docosahexanoic acid) are omega 3 derivatives and are found in most cold water fish. These fish include salmon, tuna, and mackerel. Essential fatty acids make up the outer lining or membranes of each cell. These lipid (fat) membranes determine which nutrients get into and out of the cells. They are a major component of the endoplasmic reticular detoxification membranes, nuclear membranes, and the energy producing mitochondrial membranes.

Obtaining these EFAs from the foods we eat can be challenging. Most of our foods have undergone processing that changes the essential fatty acids into toxic hydrogenated oils. The hydrogenation of the natural oils (fats) changes them into toxic trans-fatty acids.

There are receptor sites on the membranes at which point the happy hormones (neurotransmitters, serotonin and others) attach themselves. Trans-fatty acids block the cellular membrane receptor sites. A blocked or hardened cellular membrane prevents nutrients from entering and exiting the cell. The neurotransmitters (brain chemicals) are then unable to attach themselves to the cells membrane. This can lead to depression, insomnia, anxiety, fatigue, A.D.D., or any disorder that involves the brain hormones (serotonin, epinephrine, dopamine, etc.).

A deficiency of Omega-3 fat is one of the main causes of depression and other mental disorders. Omega-3 fats work to keep us mentally and emotionally strong in three ways: 1) Omega-3 fats act as precursors for the body's production of preprostaglandins and neurotransmitters (specific hormones). 2) Omega-3 fats provide the substrate for B vitamins and coenzymes to produce compounds that regulate many vital functions, including neurotransmitters. 3) Omega-3 fats provide energy and nourishment to our nerve and brain cells. Sixty percent of the US population is deficient in omega-3 fatty acids.[4]

Hunter-gatherer societies had a 1:1 or 1:5 ration of omega 6 to omega 3. Modern eating habits have change this ratio to 12:1 of omega 6 to omega 3. And this imbalance in the ratio has created an epidemic of mood disorders in America including anxiety, depression, and ADD.[5]

Longitudinal studies show that the incidence of depression has paralleled the increase of vegetable and seed oil intake (omega 6 fats). And because omega-3 fatty acids control various processes that regulate the neurotransmitters, individuals who suffer from mood disorders are consistently shown to be low in omega 3 essential fatty acids.[6] An Australian study shows that the the higher the omega 6 to omega 3 ratio, the more pronounced the symptoms of depression.[7] And low blood levels of omega 3 are a reliable marker for an increased risk of developing depression.[8]

Research shows that the countries who consume the most cold water fish—a rich source of omega 3 fats—had the lowest rate of depression and heart disease. This same researcher found that the less fish a woman consumed, the more likely she would suffer from post-partum depression.[9]

People have also responded to supplementation with omega 3 fats. Those with depression who received 1 g. daily of an omega 3 fatty acid for 12 weeks experienced a decrease in their symptoms, such as sadness, anxiety, and sleeping problems.[10]

A University of Minnesota study showed that during pregnancy, omega 3 fats decrease in a mothers blood (when compared to nonpregnant females), and stay decreased for six weeks after birth. Subsequent pregnancies made the deficiency even worse.[11] This study demonstrates the importance of omega 3 fats for fetal development. EFA is so important that the mother's brain shrinks 3% in order to provide enough DHA for fetal development.

Consider this quote from the *British Journal of Nutrition*: "Long chain fatty acid deficiency at any stage of fetal and/or infant development can result in irreversible failure to accomplish specific brain growth. There is good evidence today that lack of abundant, balanced DHA and AA in utero and infancy leads to lower intelligence quotient and visual acuity and in larger term contributes to clinical depression and attention deficit hyperactivity disorder."[12]

THE CAUSES OF EFA DEFICIENCIES

Certain groups of people have inherited a need for more EFAs and especially GLA (gamma linolenic acid) in their diet. These include individuals of Irish, Scottish, Welch, Scandinavian, Danish, British Columbian,
and Eskimo decent. Most Americans can trace their ancestry to one or
more of these groups.

There have been dramatic changes in our agricultural, food processing,
and food preparation methods in the last several decades. These changes
have created an epidemic of EFA deficiencies in most Americans.
Changes in flour-milling technology have resulted in oil rancidity and
the elimination of EFAs from most machine-processed grains.
Americans also excessively consume trans-fatty acids and hydrogenated fats in place of healthy EFAs.

One hundred years ago, our ancestors used real butter, unprocessed
grains, flax seed oil (a rich source of EFAs), and free-range cattle and
chickens. Today's farmer (in most cases, huge conglomerates like Tyson)
keeps cattle and chickens caged until death. They are fed inferior
processed grains devoid of EFAs. These farm animals are nutritiously
less efficient to human consumers. Free range cattle, chicken, and dairy
products can have over five times the amount of omega 3 and omega 6
fats in their tissues as compared to modern, industrially raised animals.

Highly processed foods are not only devoid of life-giving, health-build-
ing EFAs, but they prevent EFAs from being absorbed and effectively
utilized. Alcohol and caffeine also block conversion of EFAs to anti-
inflammatory prostaglandin hormones. And increased ingestion of toxins in our food, water, and air depletes our EFAs. The lack of breast
feeding also creates EFA deficiencies. (Omega 3 fats and DHA (docosahexanoic acid) were only recently added to infant formulas.)

SUMMARY

Excessive consumption of omega 6 fatty acids (too many vegetable oils
and grains) may interfere with the absorption of omega-3 fats. And the
excessive consumption of trans-fatty acids and hydrogenated fats interferes with EFA utilization. Poor dietary habits, including overconsump-
tion of refined sugars, caffeine, processed foods, vegetable oils, and
over-the-counter drugs, have helped create EFA deficiencies.

I encourage my patients to reduce their vegetable oil intake and increase their omega 3 fatty acid consumption. To do this, begin reducing foods processed with vegetable oils, which includes most processed snacks, crackers, chips, breads, and grain-fed livestock. Increase your omega 3 fatty acid intake by eating two or more servings of deep-sea cold-water fish each week or by supplementing with 2–6 grams of fish oil daily. To reduce the chance of having a fishy aftertaste, store your fish-oil capsules in the freezer.

Unfortunately, most deep-sea cold-water fish has been contaminated with potentially toxic mercury. Pregnant or breastfeeding mothers shouldn't eat cold-water fish at all. Other patients should use pure fish-oil capsules supplied by manufacturers who guarantee that their products are mercury free.

1.Bruno Bertozzi, et al. correspondence, *British Medical Journal,* 1996: 312: 1289-99.

2.*British Medical Journal,* 1995: 310: 1632-36

3.*British Medical Journal,* 1996: 313: 649-64

4.Galland, MD, FACN. "Leaky Gut Syndromes: Breaking the Vicious Cycle, The Third International Symposium on Functional Medicine," Vancouver, British Columbia, 1996.

5.Hibbeln JR., 1995. "Dietary polyunsaturated fatty acids and depression: when cholesterol does not satisfy."

6.Schmidt, M.A. *Smart Fats* 1997. Berkeley, CA: North Atlantic Books/Frog.

7.P.B.Adams, S. Lawson, A. Sanigorski, and A.J. Sinclair, "Arachidonic acid to eicosapentaenoic acid ratio in blood correlates positively with clinical symptoms of depression," *Lipids* 1996:31 suppl:S157-S161.

8.M.Maes et al., "Fatty acid composition in major depression; decreased omega -3 fractions in cholesteryl esters and increased C20:4 omega6/C20;5 omega 3 ratio in cholesteryl esters and phospholipids," *J Affect Disord* 1996:38:35-46.

9.J.R. Hibben, "Fish consumption and major depression," *The Lancet* 1998:351:1213.

10.*Arch Gen Psychiatry.* 2002 Oct;59(10):913-9. "A dose-ranging study of the effects of ethyl-eicosapentaenoate in patients with ongoing depression despite apparently adequate treatment with standard drugs." Peet M, Horrobin DF.

11.Holman, R.T., "The Slow Discovery of the Importance of Omega 3 essential fatty acid in Human Health." *Jour Nutr* 128 (1998) 4275-4335.

12.Broadhurst, C., Leigh, Stephen C., Cunnane, and Michael Crawford. "Rift Valley lake fish and shell fish provided brain specific nutrition for early homo." *British Jour of Nutr* 79 (1998) 3-21.

11

Food Allergies and Mood

Most people realize that food allergies can cause
wheezing, diarrhea, hives, sneezing, or a runny nose.
But the truth is that any cell, tissue, or organ (not
just the sinuses or the skin, for instance) can be
affected by a food allergy and its allergic reaction.

A*llergy* and *allergic response* are rather broad terms that describe an
illness resulting from an inflammatory reaction. The immune system mistakenly identifies a harmless substance in the environment (in this case, in food) as harmful, and it produces antibodies to attack it.

These antibodies then circulate in the blood, attached to special cells called mast cells, which are part of the immune system. The next time a person eats the food, the substance to which she is allergic (the allergen) enters the body, and attaches to the antibodies on mast cells.

The mast cells respond by releasing a host of powerful chemicals, including histamine, to "protect" the body. These chemicals produce the allergic reaction. Histamine initiates allergic inflammation, which may cause itching (hives), swelling (bronchial wheezing) or other unwanted symptoms.

I've found over the years that my patients often have several food allergies or food sensitivities (which aren't true antibody reactions) that contribute to their fatigue, depression, joint pain, muscle pain, and digestive problems.

COMMON SYMPTOMS OF FOOD ALLERGIES

- headache
- eczema
- psoriasis
- diarrhea
- colitis
- asthm
- hyperactivity

- rheumatoid arthritis
- gout
- chronic pain syndromes
- edema
- ear infections
- anxiety
- depression[1]

Unlike the classic food allergy, **food sensitivities** may not elicit an antibody reaction. Instead food sensitivities may initiate a series of bodily reactions which trigger certain bodily symptoms. These symptoms may be as innocuous as bloating, gas, or indigestion. But for some individuals, their food sensitivities trigger migraines, fatigue, mental fog, muscle or joint pain, anxiety, or depression—You may already be aware of certain foods that don't seem to "agree with you." Since these food sensitivities aren't uncovered through allergy tests, individuals may eat these illness-producing foods daily and never make the connection between their mood disorder and their diet.

Food intolerances occur from the body's inability to breakdown, digest, or assimilate a particular food.

ALLERGY TESTING

One problem is that many doctors use outdated testing and theories: specifically, the Reagin theory of allergic reactions. Around 1925, scientists in Europe discovered a substance they called Reagin. This substance appeared to be involved with allergic reactions involving the skin. Consequently, skin testing has become the primary means for determining allergies. Myopic thinking has prevented modern allergists from acknowledging that there might be another response that validates allergies, other than skin sensitivity.

Reagin was actually what we now know as immunoglobulin E (IgE), an antibody measurable through a skin prick test and the radioallergosorbent test (RAST). Both of these tests can detect acute or immediate allergic responses, but they're best for airborne allergens. They can't measure delayed sensitivity responses to food, and 95% of all food allergies occur one hour to three days after eating allergic foods. These delayed reactions must be measured using a different antibody, immunoglobulin G1-4 (IgG1-4). Many of my patients come to me having already been tested and told they had allergies. Unfortunately they were only tested for IgE antibodies. Their airborne allergies were detected, but many of their food allergies were not.

Two tests that measure immediate IgE and delayed IgG1-4 reactions are the enzyme-linked immuno-absorbent assay (ELISA) test and the food immune complex assay (FICA) test. Both offer the convenience and accuracy of measuring both types of antibodies, while costing hundreds less than RAST and skin prick tests.

All allergy tests are associated with some degree of error. Even ELISA and FICA tests are no better than 85% accurate. False positives and missed allergic foods are a common occurrence on most tests, so the gold standard for uncovering allergen sensitivities is still the one-month elimination diet. See page 123 to find out how you can conduct this diet-test for yourself. A secondary test is the pulse test. See more about this simple procedure also on page 123. For now, let's investigate the most common causes of food allergies, one by one:

CAUSES OF FOOD ALLERGIES

Cause #1: Overeating the same foods. So try to go four–five days before repeating a food; eat a varied, balanced diet.

Cause #2: Intestinal permeability. In this condition, food particles go undigested, leak across the intestinal membrane, and escape into the body. Sometimes known as "leaky gut," intestinal permeability and food allergies go hand in hand. It occurs when the lining of the digestive tract becomes permeable to toxins, which are then allowed to leak out of the digestive tract and into the bloodstream. This triggers an autoimmune reaction that can create pain and inflammation in any of the body's tissues. Persistent food allergies are usually what results.

The use of nonsteroidal anti-inflammatory drugs, steroids, antibiotics, antihistamines, caffeine, alcohol, and other prescription and nonprescription drugs renders the intestinal mucosa permeable to toxins and undigested food particles.

Find out how to treat intestinal permeability on page 121.

Cause #3: Not enough hydrochloric acid. Produced in the stomach, HCl is responsible for breaking down large foodstuff into smaller particles for entry into the small intestine. It also acts as one of the body's first lines of defense. Viruses, parasites, yeast, and bacteria are destroyed by the acidic environment produced by hydrochloric acid. Normally, adequate protein intake and a relaxed emotional state tend to increase stomach acidity.

Numerous studies have shown acid secretion declines with advancing age. The resultant rise in stomach pH (to more alkaline) can have a detrimental impact in nutrient absorption and may cause many of symptoms associated with poor health, including mood disorders. It's been estimated that 50% of Americans over the age of 60 suffer from a deficiency in hydrochloric acid.[1]

A variety of signs and symptoms can suggest decreased gastric secretions. For example, research has found 80% that of patients with achlorhydria had soreness, burning, and dryness in the mouth, and low tolerance for dentures. Thirty-four percent complained of indigestion and excessive gas. Forty percent complained of fatigue.[2]

Secretion of **gastric acid** and **pepsin** are prerequisites for optimal digestion. Gastric acid secretion is a fundamental process in assuring proper digestion and absorption. Gastric acid secretions are responsible for stimulating the release of pancreatic enzymes. A deficiency of hydrochloric stomach acid triggers a chain reaction of digestive disorders. Without enough stomach acid to stimulate pancreatic enzyme production, further digestion and absorption in the small intestine is compromised, and this leads to malabsorption problems.

Without adequate gastric secretions, foods may be incompletely digested and may subsequently be absorbed into the bloodstream. Acidic stomach pH also impacts absorption of selected vitamins, minerals, amino acids, and other nutrients. Low stomach acid can decrease the absorption of calcium, folic acid, iron, vitamin B12, vitamin D, and zinc. A deficiency in any of these may trigger poor immune function, anxiety, fatigue, depression, and pain.

Here is a list of some of the symptoms associated with low stomach acid (achlorhydria).[3]

- bloating
- gas
- indigestion
- heartburn
- distention after eating
- diarrhea
- constipation
- hair loss in women
- parasitic infections

- rectal itching
- malaise
- multiple food allergies
- nausea
- nausea after taking supplements
- restless legs
- sore or burning tongue
- dry mouth

Cause #4: Not enough pancreatic enzymes. One of the pancreas's most important functions is to supply an adequate amount of enzymes to aid in digestion. These enzymes breakdown foodstuff and allow the smaller molecules and nutrients to be absorbed into the bloodstream. They include trypsin, amylase, lipase, chymotrypsin, and carboxypeptidase. Amylase reduces large chains of starch polypeptides to smaller disaccharides, and lipase is the fat-digesting enzyme.

Enzymes, essential for proper digestion, may become deficient for a variety of reasons including age and poor diet (excess sugar, processed food, deficient essential fatty acids, trans-fatty acids, overeating, etc.).

Raw, unprocessed foods contain their own digestive enzymes. When we eat these foods, we spare our own pancreatic enzymes. Eating processed foods, on the other hand, requires our body to secrete extra amounts of pancreatic enzymes. Over time, processed foods deplete a persons own pancreatic enzyme stores.

Since they help so much for digestion, these enzymes help regulate many of the inflammatory reactions in the body. One of the substances capable of eliciting such an inflammatory reaction are hormones known as kinins. Triggered by allergic foods or chemicals, kinins are capable of causing severe and painful inflammatory reactions. Inflammation can occur anywhere kinins are present, including the brain. This can lead to brain fog, anxiety and or depression. Proteolytic enzymes are able to reduce the number of kinins and therefore prevent the inflammatory reactions associated with hormones.

Low-fat (which are often low-protein) and starvation diets, along with deficient hydrochloric acid, pepsinogen, or digestive enzymes can create amino-acid deficiencies. Remember that amino acids are what create the neurotransmitters. Well, proteolytic enzymes are also built from amino acids. So…no amino acids, no inflammatory/pain blocking proteolytic enzymes.

Malabsorption issues and the nutritional deficiencies they create are perhaps the greatest culprits in the fight against inflammation. This is why I recommend that patients hedge their bets (even if they're not having digestive problems) and take digestive enzymes. All patients over the age of 35—or with chronic health problems—should take digestive enzymes, even if they're not currently suffering from a digestive illness.

You should be having at least one bowel movement every 24 hours. Having a bowel movement after each meal is optimal. Notice how often your pets have a bowel movement…after every meal. Having three or more bowel movements in a day can seem like a lot when you were, until recently, having only one every few days. But I assure you; it's healthy. I recommend my patients use a potent pancreatic digestive enzyme formula that utilizes USP porcine-derived high-potency pancreatin for reliable and consistent enzyme activity.

Cause #5: Intestinal dysbiosis. The intestinal tract contains hundreds of microorganisms (bacteria and yeast) that normally don't cause any health problems. However, when the intestinal tract is repetitively exposed to toxic substances (antibiotics, steroids, anti-inflammatory medications, etc.) these microorganisms (yeast and bad bacteria) begin to proliferate and create an imbalance in the bowel flora. This is known as intestinal dysbiosis.

The intestinal tract contains some 2–3 lbs. of bacteria. The GI tract contains approximately 100,000 billion viable bacteria. The skin harbors approximately 1,000 billion viable bacteria. There are a total of 10,000 billion cells in the body. As you can see, there are more of them (bacteria) than there are of us (human cells). When normal healthy intestinal bacteria levels are depleted, a person becomes more susceptible to disease. For instance, the infective dose of Salmonella enteritidis decreases from 100,000 to approximately 10. Dysbiosis can be treated with probiotics, which can be found at healthfood stores. *Lactobacillus* (acidophilus, casei, and rhamnosus) and *Bifido bacterium bifidum* are the two most important probiotics.

TREATING INTESTINAL PERMEABILITY

Intestinal permeability can be measured by using a special functional-medicine test available from Great Smokies Laboratory. (See Appendix

B.) But if you suspect you have intestinal permeability, take the following steps:

- **Take three probiotic capsules daily** on an empty stomach for two months.

- **Start supplementing hydrochloric acid with pepsin.**

- **Immediately begin an elimination diet** to pinpoint any food allergies. Pay particular attention to gluten, a protein found in most grains, because it can be very irritating to the intestinal lining.

- **Make sure you're taking fish oil,** 1,000–2,000 mg. daily. The omega 3 fatty acids in fish oil help repair the intestinal tract. They also help reduce inflammation associated with leaky gut. One study showed that 2.7 grams daily put Crohn's disease patients into remission.[4]

For additional supplementation, I recommend a product especially developed for intestinal permeability called Leaky Gut Formula. (See Appendix B for ordering information.) Dosage is six capsules daily, best taken between meals in divided doses, for one–two months. Leaky Gut Formula should be taken along with the elimination diet outlined below. It contains all the essential nutrients to help correct intestinal permeability:

- **Large amounts (6,000 mg.) of the amino acid glutamine,** the primary fuel for intestinal cell function, are included to meet the high energy demands of the GI tract, liver, and immune system during periods of physiological stress. Glutamine also transports potentially toxic ammonia concentrations to the kidneys for excretion. Intestinal uptake of glutamine accounts for 40% of total body uptake, and chronic intestinal insults from xenotoxins (NSAIDs, antibiotics, etc.) create a shortage of glutamine.
- **Acacia** contributes soluble, non-bulking fiber that is readily fermentable into acetic, butyric, and propionic short-chain fatty acids that create a supportive environment for growth of beneficial Lactobacillus bacteria, assist water absorption, and support colonic cell function.
- **Nutraflora FOS** supplies non-digestible fructooligosaccharides to further encourage growth of beneficial microorganisms.
- **N-acetyl-D-glucosamine** is used as a structural component of intestinal mucous secretions that protect intestinal tissues and help food pass through the GI tract.

THE ELIMINATION DIET

If you suspect you have intestinal permeability or food allergies, I recommend you follow the elimination diet according to these guidelines:

1. For one month, eliminate:
- all dairy products (except butter) including milk, cheese, yogurt, and ice cream.
- all corn and related products: corn syrup, popcorn etc.
- all gluten products, including wheat, oats, barley, kamut, spelt, and all flours.
- all soy products.
- all nightshade foods, including white potatoes, peppers, tomatoes, tobacco, and eggplant. Nightshades contain a poison similar to belladonna that may cause muscle or joint pain.
- all caffeinated foods (see page 74 for guidance on this).

- **After one month, start to reintroduce** one item from one eliminated food group at a time. The day of the challenge, eat a few servings of the eliminated food group (Wheat: pasta, toast, crackers, bread, etc.) then wait three days and reintroduce another food group (Dairy: milk, cheese, ice cream, etc.) and again, eat a few servings. If after three days of challenging a food group, there's no associated negative reaction (headaches, stomach pain, bloating, runny nose, congestion, muscle or joint pain, low moods, fatigue, heaviness, etc.) then start to slowly add these items back into the regular diet.

- **Listen carefully to your body.** If you experience a negative reaction to any food within three days of challenging a specific group, you should discontinue that particular food group for another month and then repeat the process.

- **Protect from future damage.** Try to avoid all NSAIDs, including Advil, Motrin, etc. If you need antibiotics, then take probiotics (take them 12 hours apart) as well.

THE PULSE SELF-TEST

The forbidden foods listed in the elimination diet guidelines are by far the most common allergic foods. However, practically any food can trigger an allergic reaction. For this reason, you might want to dig a little deeper to pinpoint sensitivities to specific foods. Foods can actually be tested by merely tasting them. If a food elicits a rise in resting pulse rate, this indicates an allergic reaction. This is because the pulse is controlled by the autonomic nervous system, and stress causes this system to increase blood flow and pulse rate.

To use the pulse test, first follow the elimination diet for one month. If you want to get started pulse-testing sooner, try instead a one- or two-day modified fast: allowable foods include filtered water, diluted fruit juice (2/3 water), watermelon, cantaloupe, bananas, brown-rice, and lamb.

Then determine your resting pulse rate: count your pulse for a full minute while sitting still. (Sites commonly used to check the pulse are the underside of the wrist and the neck near the Adam's apple). Your resting pulse is the pulse consistently found before eating, or an average of the lowest pulses most commonly recorded.

To get the most accurate baseline reading:

1. **Take your pulse** in bed before rising, before breakfast, after breakfast, in the middle of the morning, before lunch, after lunch, in the middle of the afternoon, before dinner, after dinner, in the middle of the evening, and before bed.

2. **Keep a food diary,** record your pulse rates and any symptoms, and compare them to your resting pulse rate. Does a pattern emerge? If there is no consistent pattern, there may be too many interfering substances undermining the process.

3. **Try the elimination diet** for four–five days. Along with the obvious elimination foods, foods or chemicals in question should also be avoided during this time.

To test individual foods:

1. **While sitting quietly, take your pulse.**

2. **Then challenge this pulse** by chewing a small amount of food or food supplement (don't swallow) for a full minute. Liquids can be held and swished around in the mouth.

3. **After one minute, take your pulse** for a full minute.

4. **At the end of this time, expel the substance,** and rinse out your mouth with pure water, which should also be expelled.

5. **Take your pulse again.** If it returns to the resting value, you can repeat the process with another substance.

A positive-reaction food or supplement will elevate the pulse above six points. Avoid all these foods for two–three months. If other symptoms occur after testing, such as headache, sore throat, or fuzzy thinking, this is a severe positive, and the food should be avoided for three–six months.

All reactive foods should be reintroduced slowly, one at a time, and not more than one in a month's time. If you continue to have reactions to reintroduced allergic foods, avoid them again for three months before retesting.

TREATING (LOW STOMACH ACID)

Numerous studies have shown that acid secretion declines with advancing age. It's been estimated that 50% of Americans over the age of 60 suffer from achlorhydria, a deficiency in hydrochloric acid. The resulting rise in stomach pH can cause many of the symptoms associated with food allergies and other symptoms of poor health.

Low stomach acid may also cause the very same symptoms associated with GERD. Unless you've had an upper GI endoscopy, biopsy, or blood test that shows a definitive case of GERD or *H.pylori,* then you may not have GERD at all and you may be causing more problems by using antacid medications.

We need gastric acid and pepsin for optimal digestion of food, absorption of nutrients, and release of pancreatic enzymes. An HCl deficiency triggers a chain reaction of digestive disorders, including malabsorption. Foods may be incompletely digested and subsequently absorbed into the bloodstream, where they can lead to food allergies, triggering pain and inflammation throughout the body.

That's why antacids can be so dangerous for those who don't really need them! First, the esophageal sphincter is stimulated to close by the release of stomach acids. When there's not enough stomach acid present—because antacids have neutralized them—the esophageal sphincter may not close properly. This allows acid to travel back up into the esophagus and cause heartburn, also called esophageal reflux or gastroesophageal reflux disease—GERD. GERD is usually treated by antacids, but antacids *could* make the GERD worse.

Second, the stomach needs an acidic environment for HCl to turn the enzyme pepsinogen into pepsin. No acid equals no pepsin, which is needed for digestion, especially protein. No protein digestion means no amino acids. No amino acids, no neurotansmitters (serotonin, dopamine, norepinephrine, etc.).

Last, an acidic environment is one of the body's first lines of defense, destroying viruses, parasites, yeast, and bacteria. So if you're suffering from heartburn, try the solutions below rather than antacids.

- **Take a pancreatic digestive enzyme** with each meal. If you've been taking Nexium, Prevacid, Pepcid, Prevpac, Prilosec, Propulsid, Reglan, or Zantac for over three months, then you may have to stay on the medications along with taking digestive enzymes. Many of my patients have found that they don't need these prescription medications once they start taking a good high-potency digestive enzyme like the one I use in my practice.

- **If you continue to have problems with reflux** even after taking digestive enzymes, then try taking Betaine (HCl) with pepsin, which is available from your healthfood store.* And always take pancreatic enzymes along with HCl. Follow the guidelines below for use.

1. Take one capsule containing 600–650 mg. of Betaine HCl along with 100–200 mg. of pepsin at the beginning of your next meal. Continue taking one capsule with each meal for the next five days.

2. After five days, increase your dose to two capsules with each meal. Continue this for five days

3. Now its time to start increasing your dose by one capsule each day until you feel a sense of warmth, fullness, or other odd sensation in your stomach not normally experienced. This sensation probably indicates that you've taken more HCl than you need. If so simply reduce your dose by one capsule at your next meal. It's recommended you don't take more than five (600–650 mg.) capsules at a time.

4. Once you've established a dose (five capsules or fewer), continue this dose at meals.

5. It is common that, as your stomach regains the ability to produce an adequate concentration of HCl, you will require fewer capsules.

---

*I don't recommend HCL if you have been diagnosed with a peptic ulcer, because HCL can irritate sensitive tissue. It can also corrode teeth, so capsules should not be emptied into food or beverages.

6. With smaller meals, you may wish to reduce your dosage.

Individuals with low HCl/pepsin typically don't respond as well to botanicals and supplements, so, to maximize the absorption and benefits to the nutrients prescribed, it's important to be consistent with your HCl/pepsin supplementation.

OTHER NATURAL REMEDIES

1. Supplement with Inflammation Formula: I often recommend my "Inflammation Formula: to my patients to help reduce allergy symptoms. The formula contains the following:

• **Tumeric root** extract inhibits enzymes associated with some inflammatory hormones.
• **Rosemary leaf extract** helps block the causes of some allergic reactions.
• **Holy basil leaf extract** helps boost natural anti-inflammatory chemicals.
• **Green tea leaf extract** is a potent antioxidant that increases the body's own anti-inflammatory activity.
• **Ginger root extract** reduces inflammation and helps regulate inflammatory systems.
• **Chinese goldenthread root, barberry root extract, and baikal skullcap root extract** reduce inflammatory chemicals.
• **Protykin polygonum cuspidatum extract** is a potent antioxidant and reduces inflammatory chemicals.

2. Supplement with extra vitamin C. It's a natural antihistamine and may reduce the symptoms associated with allergic reactions. Take up to bowel tolerance.

3. Supplement with stinging nettle root, which helps reduce allergic rhinitis (runny nose) and hay fever symptoms. It also helps prevent the bronchial spasms associated with asthma. Take 500–1,000 mg. three times daily.

4. Supplement with quercetin, a bioflavonoid (plant pigment) found in black tea, blue-green algae, broccoli, onions, red apples, and red wine. It inhibits the synthesis of certain enzymes responsible for triggering allergic reactions. It is chemically similar to the allergy prevention medication Cromolyn. Take 500–1,000 twice daily. It may take months before quercetin reaches its peak of effectiveness. It can interfere with the absorption of certain antibiotics, so don't take quercetin and antibiotics together.

5. Supplement with methylsulfonylmethane (MSM), a natural organic sulfur compound found in plant and animal tissues. MSM has proven beneficial in the treatment of allergic and inflammation disorders. It provides sulfur, an essential component in detoxification. Due to its strong anti-inflammatory properties, it's included in our Essential Therapeutics Arthritis Formula. Normal dosage is 500 mg. three–four times daily.

6. Supplement with Boswellia serrata (Indian frankincense), an Indian herb with anti-inflammatory properties. It helps prevent allergic inflammation and can be used to treat allergies and arthritis. Take 200 mg. three times daily.

7. Reduce grains and other high–omega-6 foods. Omega-6 foods produce arachidonic acid, which leads to more inflammatory chemicals.

8. Increase fish oil (omega-3) consumption to 2,000–9,000 mg. daily. Omega-3s reduce inflammation.

1. Vellas B, Balas D, Albarde JL. "Effects of aging process on digestive functions." *Comprehensive Therapy* 1991;17(8):46-52

2. This is cited in *Alternative Medicine Review,* Volume 2, No. 2, March, 1997. Sharp GS, Fister HW. "The diagnosis and treatment of achlorhydria 10 year study." *Journal of American Geriatric Society,* 1967; 15; 786-791.

3. Great Smokies Laboratory *Functional Assessment Resource Manual* Fall 1999: G-5.

4. Belluz A. Brignola C, Campieri Met al. "Effects of an enteric-coated fish oil preparation on relapses in Crohn's disease." *N. Engl J Med* 1996;334:1557-60

┌─────┐
│ 12 │
└─────┘

A Summary of Your Step-by-Step Plan

There is a lot of information to absorb in this book. I've tried to keep the material simple, focusing on the most important points. Even so, you may be feeling overwhelmed. Take heart; you're gonna treat this thing, and *beat* this thing, one step at a time.

1. **Don't stop taking your prescription antidepressant.** Wait until after you've been using my recommendations below and when you're feeling stronger, healthier in general, working with your doctor, slowly wean off you're prescription antidepressant (if you wish) over a period of two-three months

2. **Start taking an ODA multivitamin/mineral formula** along with a minimum of two grams of fish oil, and free form amino acids.

3. **Complete the Brain Function Profile,** and follow my advice in chapter 5 on starting amino acid replacement therapy. Individuals with breakthrough anxiety should begin taking inositol in addition.

4. **Sleep tight.** Make sure you're consistently going into deep restorative sleep each night. If not, follow my advice in the chapter on sleep disorders.

5. Test for adrenal fatigue. If the test is positive, take the steps outlined in chapter 7 to reduce your stress and rebuild your stress-coping adrenal glands.

6. Get a pill book from your library or bookstore, and read about all the prescription drugs you're taking. Make sure that none of these drugs is contributing to your depression.

7. Start or maintain an exercise program.

8. Use St. John's Wort along with your amino-acid replacement therapy, if needed.

9. Clean up your diet. Eat three meals a day or several small meals. Reduce your intake of omega-6 vegetable oils and avoid all processed foods. Increase your intake of whole foods.

10. Spend 30–60 minutes a day reading uplifting material such as the Bible or other religious texts, Wayne Dyer, Norman Vincent Peale, or your favorite comic. Pray, meditate, or just spend time alone with your thoughts. Remember that our thoughts create our feelings, and our feelings create the state of our health. Happy thoughts create happy feelings, and happy feelings create happy and healthy molecules, cells, organs, minds, and bodies. Negative, depressed thoughts create negative, depressed feelings and unhealthy minds and bodies.

Controlling our thoughts is difficult even when we aren't suffering from depression or anxiety. However, once you begin to build up your stress-coping savings account, you'll have the mental strength to start observing and eventually controlling your thoughts. This is what your hour of power is for: time to think, feel, observe, and when needed, change any unwanted negative thought patterns.

The first step to beating anxiety and depression is to love yourself. The power that created, from two cells, the trillions of cells we call a human being, is still within you. This incredible miracle that you've become is unique and special. Find yourself. Forgive yourself. Love yourself. Find your purpose. Help others less fortunate. Happiness is contagious, once you catch a glimmer of it, pass it on.

Appendix A
Brain Function Questionnaire

Check each of the sentences below that applies to you.

__ Your life seems incomplete.
__ You feel shy with all but your closest friends.
__ You have feelings of insecurity.
__ You often feel unequal to others.
__ When things go right, you feel undeserving.
__ You feel something is missing in your life.
__ You occasionally feel a low self-worth or -esteem.
__ You feel inadequate as a person.
__ You frequently feel fearful when there is nothing to fear.

If three or more of these descriptions apply to your present feelings, you are probably part of the "O" group. Read about a deficiency of opioid neurotransmitters on page 39.

Check each of the sentences below that applies to you.

__ You often feel anxious for no reason.
__ You sometimes feel "free-floating" anxiety.
__ You frequently feel "edgy," and it's difficult to relax.
__ You often feel a "knot" in your stomach.
__ Falling asleep is sometimes difficult.
__ It's hard to turn your mind off when you want to relax.
__ You occasionally experience feelings of panic for no reason.
__ You often use alcohol or other sedatives to calm down.

If three or more of these descriptions apply to your present feelings, you are probably part of the "G" group. Read about a deficiency of GABA on page 40.

Check each of the sentences below that applies to you.

___ You lack pleasure in life.
___ You feel there are no real rewards in life.
___ You have unexplained lack of concern for others, even loved ones.
___ You experience decreased parental feelings.
___ Life seems less "colorful" or "flavorful."
___ Things that used to be "fun" just aren't any longer.
___ You have become a less spiritual or socially concerned person.

If three or more of these descriptions apply to your present feelings, you are probably part of the "D" group. Read about a deficiency of dopamine on page 42.

Check each of the sentences below that applies to you.

___ You suffer from a lack of energy.
___ You often find it difficult to "get going."
___ You suffer from decreased drive.
___ You often start projects and then don't finish them.
___ You frequently feel a need to sleep or "hibernate."
___ You feel depressed a good deal of the time.
___ You occasionally feel paranoid.
___ Your survival seems threatened.
___ You are bored a great deal of the time.

If three or more of these descriptions apply to your present feelings, you are probably part of the "N" group. Read about a deficiency of norepinephrine on page 43.

Check each of the sentences below that applies to you.

___ It's hard for you to go to sleep.

___ You can't stay asleep.

___ You often find yourself irritable.

___ Your emotions often lack rationality.

___ You occasionally experience unexplained tears.

___ Noise bothers you more than it used to; it seems louder than normal.

___ You flare up at others more easily than you used to; you experience unprovoked anger.

___ You feel depressed much of the time.

___ You find you are more susceptible to pain.

___ You prefer to be left alone.

If three or more of these descriptions apply to your present feelings, you are probably part of the "S" group. Read about a deficiency of serotonin on page 45.

Appendix B

Resources

To contact Dr. Murphree:
1-205-879-2383
(toll-free) 1-888-884-9577
3401 Independence Drive suite 121
Birmingham AL 35209
www.TreatingAndBeating.com

Supplements, tests, and literature
To order any of these products, or for a free catalog featuring the entire *Essential Therapeutics* line, call 1-888-884-9577 or visit us on the web at www.Treatingandbeating.com

Supplements available for purchase from Dr. Murphree
- **Complete Multivitamin/mineral Formula with digestive enzymes and fish oil**: 60 packs per bottle
- **Basic optimal daily allowance multivitamin/mineral:** 180 tablets
- **5HTP** 50 mg. and 100 mg. capsules available; guaranteed to be "peak x" free
- **L-Phenylalanine:** 500 mg. capsules
- **DL-Phenylalanine:** 500 mg. capsules
- **GABA:** 500 mg. capsules
- **L-Theonine:** 100 mg. capsules
- **SAMe:** 200 mg. 30 blister packs per box
- **St. John's Wort:** standardized to .3 Hypercin and 300 mg. per capsule
- **Ginkgo biloba**
- **Inflammation formula**
- **Free-form amino acids**
- **Leaky Gut Formula**
- **Digestive enzymes**
- **Fish oil** (mercury free)
- **Sublingual DHEA:** 5 mg. and 25 mg.
- **Sublingual melatonin:** 3 mg.
- **Sublingual timed-release melatonin:** 3 mg.
- **Adrenal cortex**
- **GTA Forte** thyroid supplement

Books by Dr. Murphree
• *Treating and Beating Fibromyalgia and Chronic Fatigue Syndrome.*
• *Heart Disease: What Your Doctor Won't Tell You.*
• *Treating and Beating Fibromyalgia and Chronic Fatigue Syndrome:
A Patient Self-Help Manual.*

Testing Resources
(Tests require a referral from Dr. Murphree or your physician before
you can order.)

Neuroscience: 1-888-342-7272 or www.neuroscience.com
• urine-based tests that reveal amino-acid deficiencies and resulting
neurotransmitter depletion.
• tests for serotonin, dopamine, GABA, and epinephrine.

Great Smokies Labs: 1-800-522-4762 or www.gsdl.com
• adrenal cortex profile shows cortisol and DHEA levels
• food allergy testing
• melatonin profile test

Information Resources
www.orthomolecular.org
Orthomolecular Development
3100 N. Hillside,
Wichita, KS 67219
316-682-3100

Journal of Orthomolecular Medicine
16 Florence Avenue
Toronto, Ontario, Canada M2N-1E9
1-416-723-2117
(supplies names of orthomolecular physicians)

American Holistic Medical Association (AHMA)
4101 Boone Trail
Raleigh, NC 27607
1-703-261-2101

American College for Advancement in Medicine (ACAM)
23121 Verdugo Drive Suite 204
P.O. Box 3427
Laguna Hills, CA 92654
1-949-583-7666

American Association of Naturopathic Physicians
601 Valley, Suite 105
Seattle, WA 98109
1-206-298-0125
www.naturopathic.org

American Academy of Environmental Medicine (AAEM)
P.O. Box CN 1001-8001
New Hope, PA 18938
1-316-684-5500

Orthomolecular Medical Associations Around the World
UNITED STATES OF AMERICA
Society for Orthomolecular Health Medicine (OHM)
President: Richard Kunin, MD
2698 Pacific Avenue, San Francisco, CA 94115
Tel: 415 922 6462
Fax: 415 346 2519
sohma@aol.com

UNITED KINGDOM
Institute for Optimum Nutrition (ION)
Contact: Adam Porter-Blake
Blades Court, Deodar Road, London SW15 2NU
Tel: 44 208 877 9993
Fax: 44 208 877 9980
reception@ion.ac.uk
www.ion.ac.uk

ARGENTINA
Sociedad Argentina de Medicina Integrada Ortomolecular
President: Alberto Dardanelli, MD
Vuelta de Obligado 3046, 6o. piso, 1429 Buenos Aires
Tel/Fax: 54 11 4703 4252
imointernational@hotmail.com
www.acmed.com.ar

AUSTRALIA
Orthomolecular Medical Association of Australia (OMMA)
President: Dr. Ian Brighthope
13 Hilton Street, Beaumaris, Victoria 3193
Tel: 61 3 9589 6088
Fax: 61 3 9589 5158
mail@acnem.org
www.acnem.org

SOMA Health Association of Australia
Secretary: J.M. Sulima
P.O. Box 915, Leichardt NSW 2040
Tel: 61 2 9789 4805
Fax: 61 2 9922 5747
help@soma-health.com.au
www.soma-health.com.au

BELGIUM
Belgian Society for Orthomolecular Medicine
Vlaams Instituut voor Orthomoleculaire Wetenschappen (VIOW)
Contact: Werner A. Fache, MD
Kerkstraat 101, 9270 Laarne
Tel: 32 9 222 2400
Fax: 32 9 366 1838
werner.fache@planetinternet.be; walter.fache@viow.be
www.viow.be

BRAZIL
Brazilian Society for Orthomolecular Medicine
Sociedade Brasileira de Medicina Ortomolecular (SBMO)
President: Oslim Malina, MD
Rua 7 Abril, 813, Curtiba 80040 PR
Tel/Fax: 55 41 264 8034

CANADA
Canadian Society for Orthomolecular Medicine (CSOM)
Secretary: Steven Carter
16 Florence Avenue, Toronto, ON M2N 1E9
Tel: 416 733 2117
Fax: 416 733 2352
centre@orthomed.org
www.orthomed.org

DENMARK
Danish Society for Orthomolecular Medicine
Dansk Selskab for Orthomolekylaer Medicin (DSOM)
President: Claus Hancke, MD
Lyngby Hovedgade 37, DK 2800 Kgs. Lyngby
Tel: 45 45 88 0900
Fax: 45 45 88 0947
ch@iom.dk

GERMANY
German Society for Orthomolecular Medicine
Deutsche Gesellschaft fur Orthomolekulare Medizin (DGOM)
SittardstraBe 21, 41061 Monchengladbach
Tel: 49 21 6120 9729
Fax: 49 21 6118 2290

Munchner Gesellschaft zur Forderung der Orthomolekulare
Medizin e. V. (GOMM)
Zur Bergwiese 7, 82152 Planegg
Tel: 49 89 8959 0105
Fax: 49 89 8982 6598

ITALY
Italian Society for Orthomolecular Medicine
Associazione Internationale di Medicina Ortomolecolare (AIMO)
President: Adolfo Panfili, MD
Via Della Mendola, 68, 00135 Rome
Tel: 39 06 331 5961
Fax: 39 06 331 5943
panfili@aimo.it
www.aimo.it

KOREA
Korean Society for Orthomolecular Medicine (KSOM)
President: Sung Ho Park, PhD
Bupyong-Dong 199-20
Bupyong-Gu 403-821 Incheon
ksom@ksom.or.kr
www.ksom.or.kr

MEXICO
Mexican Society for Orthomolecular Medicine
Sociedad de Medicina Ortomolecular
President: Hector E. Solorzano, MD
Los Aipes No. 1024, Col. Independencia, 44340 Guadalajara, Jal.
Tel: 52 3 651 5476
Fax: 52 3 637 0030
hector@solorzano.com

THE NETHERLANDS
Dutch Society for Orthomolecular Medicine
Maatschappij ter Bevordering van de Orthomoleccaire
Geneeskunde (MBOG)
Contact: F.J.A. Eissens-van Goor
Zuiderstraat 4, 9479 PP Noordlaren
Tel: 31 50 409 2717
Fax: 31 50 409 2738
secretariaat@mbog.nl
www.mbog.nl

SPAIN
Sociedad Espanola de Medicina Ortomolecular
Pres: Luis Arnaiz Duro de Paradis
Balmes 412 08022-Barcelona
Tel: 34 93 254 6000 Fax: 34 93 254 4774
www.ortomolecular.com

SWITZERLAND
Swiss Society for Nutritional Healing and Orthomolecular
Medicine
Fachgesellschaft fur Emahrungsheikunde und
Orthomolekularmedizin Schweiz
President: John van Limburg Stirum, MD
Spruengli-Weg 9, CH-8802 Kilchberg
Tel: 41 1 715 6401
Fax: 41 1 715 6403
info@feos.ch
www.feos.ch

Index